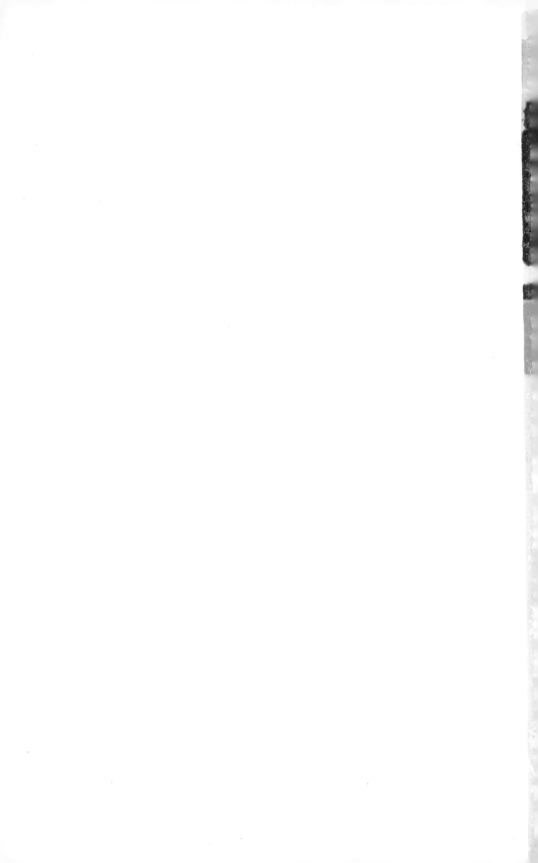

PAIN MEDICINE
A CASE-BASED LEARNING SERIES

The Hip and Pelvis

Other books in this series:

 The Spine
9780323756365

 The Shoulder and Elbow
9780323758772

 The Knee
9780323762588

 Headache and Facial Pain
9780323834568

 The Wrist and Hand
9780323834537

 The Chest Wall and Abdomen
9780323846882

 The Ankle and Foot
9780323870382

PAIN MEDICINE
A CASE-BASED LEARNING SERIES

The Hip and Pelvis

STEVEN D. WALDMAN, MD, JD

ELSEVIER

Elsevier
1600 John F. Kennedy Blvd.
Ste 1800
Philadelphia, PA 19103-2899

PAIN MEDICINE: A CASE-BASED LEARNING SERIES   ISBN: 978-0-323-76297-7
THE HIP AND PELVIS

Notice

Practitioners and researchers must always rely on their own experience and knowledge in evaluating and using any information, methods, compounds or experiments described herein. Because of rapid advances in the medical sciences, in particular, independent verification of diagnoses and drug dosages should be made. To the fullest extent of the law, no responsibility is assumed by Elsevier, authors, editors or contributors for any injury and/or damage to persons or property as a matter of products liability, negligence or otherwise, or from any use or operation of any methods, products, instructions, or ideas contained in the material herein.

Library of Congress Control Number: 2021936696

Executive Content Strategist: Michael Houston
Content Development Specialist: Jeannine Carrado/Laura Klien
Director, Content Development: Ellen Wurm-Cutter
Publishing Services Manager: Shereen Jameel
Senior Project Manager: Karthikeyan Murthy
Design Direction: Amy Buxton

Printed in The United States of America.

Last digit is the print number: 9 8 7 6 5 4 3 2 1

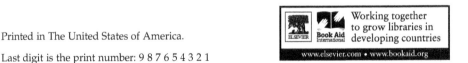

Working together to grow libraries in developing countries

www.elsevier.com • www.bookaid.org

It's Harder Than It Looks
MAKING THE CASE FOR CASE-BASED LEARNING

For sake of full disclosure, I was one of those guys. You know, the ones who wax poetic about how hard it is to teach our students how to do procedures. Let me tell you, teaching folks how to do epidurals on women in labor certainly takes its toll on the coronary arteries. It's true, I am amazing. . .I am great. . .I have nerves of steel. Yes, I could go on like this for hours. . .but you have heard it all before. But, it's again that time of year when our new students sit eagerly before us, full of hope and dreams. . .and that harsh reality comes slamming home. . .it is a lot harder to teach beginning medical students "doctoring" than it looks.

A few years ago, I was asked to teach first-year medical and physician assistant students how to take a history and perform a basic physical exam. In my mind I thought "this should be easy. . .no big deal". I won't have to do much more than show up. After all, I was the guy who wrote that amazing book on physical diagnosis. After all, I had been teaching medical students, residents, and fellows how to do highly technical (and dangerous, I might add) interventional pain management procedures since right after the Civil War. Seriously, it was no big deal...I could do it in my sleep. . .with one arm tied behind my back. . .blah. . .blah. . .blah.

For those of you who have had the privilege of teaching "doctoring," you already know what I am going to say next. *It's harder than it looks!* Let me repeat this to disabuse any of you who, like me, didn't get it the first time. *It is harder than it looks!* I only had to meet with my first-year medical and physician assistant students a couple of times to get it through my thick skull: **It really is harder than it looks**. In case you are wondering, the reason that our students look back at us with those blank, confused, bored, and ultimately dismissive looks is simple: They lack context. That's right, they lack the context to understand what we are talking about.

It's really that simple. . .or hard. . .depending on your point of view or stubbornness, as the case may be. To understand why context is king, you have to look only as far as something as basic as the Review of Systems. The Review of Systems is about as basic as it gets, yet why is it so perplexing to our students? Context. I guess it should come as no surprise to anyone that the student is completely lost when you talk about. . .let's say. . .the "constitutional" portion of the Review of Systems, without the context of what a specific constitutional finding, say a fever or chills, might mean to a patient who is suffering from the acute onset of headaches. If you tell the student that you need to ask about fever, chills, and the other "constitutional" stuff and you take it no further, you might as well be talking about the

International Space Station. Just save your breath; it makes absolutely no sense to your students. Yes, they want to please, so they will memorize the elements of the Review of Systems, but that is about as far as it goes. On the other hand, if you present the case of Jannette Patton, a 28-year-old first-year medical resident with a fever and headache, you can see the lights start to come on. By the way, this is what Jannette looks like, and as you can see, Jannette is sicker than a dog. This, at its most basic level, is what *Case-Based Learning* is all about.

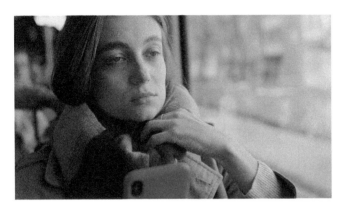

I would like to tell you that, smart guy that I am, I immediately saw the light and became a convert to *Case-Based Learning*. But truth be told, it was COVID-19 that really got me thinking about *Case-Based Learning*. Before the COVID-19 pandemic, I could just drag the students down to the med/surg wards and walk into a patient room and riff. Everyone was a winner. For the most part, the patients loved to play along and thought it was cool. The patient and the bedside was all I needed to provide the context that was necessary to illustrate what I was trying to teach—the why headache and fever don't mix kind of stuff. Had COVID-19 not rudely disrupted my ability to teach at the bedside, I suspect that you would not be reading this *Preface*, as I would not have had to write it. Within a very few days after the COVID-19 pandemic hit, my days of bedside teaching disappeared, but my students still needed context. This got me focused on how to provide the context they needed. The answer was, of course, *Case-Based Learning*. What started as a desire to provide context. . .because it really was **harder than it looked**. . .led me to begin work on this eight-volume *Case-Based Learning* textbook series. What you will find within these volumes are a bunch of fun, real-life cases that help make each patient come alive for the student. These cases provide the contextual teaching points that make it easy for the teacher to explain why, when Jannette's chief complaint is, *"My head is killing me and I've got a fever,"* it is a big deal.

Have fun!

Steven D. Waldman, MD, JD
Spring 2021

A very special thanks to my editors, Michael Houston PhD, Jeannine Carrado, and Karthikeyan Murthy, for all of their hard work and perseverance in the face of disaster. Great editors such as Michael, Jeannine, and Karthikeyan make their authors look great, for they not only understand how to bring the Three Cs of great writing. . .Clarity + Consistency + Conciseness. . .to the author's work, but unlike me, they can actually punctuate and spell!

Steven D. Waldman, MD, JD

P.S. . . .Sorry for all the ellipses, guys!

CONTENTS

1

Addie Brooks

A 52-Year-Old Woman With Right Hip and Groin Pain

- Learn the common causes of hip pain.
- Develop an understanding of the unique anatomy of the hip joint.
- Develop an understanding of the causes of hip joint arthritis.
- Learn the clinical presentation of osteoarthritis of the hip joint.
- Learn how to use physical examination to identify pathology of the hip joint.
- Develop an understanding of the treatment options for osteoarthritis of the hip joint.
- Learn the appropriate testing options to help diagnose osteoarthritis of the hip joint.
- Learn to identify red flags waving in patients who present with hip pain.
- Develop an understanding of the role in interventional pain management in the treatment of hip pain.

Addie Brooks

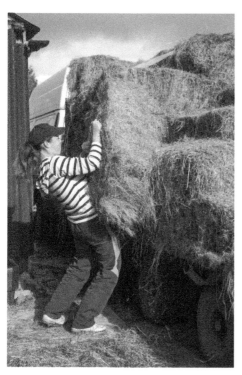

Addie Brooks is a 52-year-old rancher with the chief complaint of, "I've got a hitch in my git-along." Addie went on to say that she wouldn't have bothered coming in, but "it is coming up on calving season and those cows gotta eat." I asked Addie if anything like this has happened before. She shook her head and said, "You can't run cattle and not have something aching or paining. But this hitch is really wearing me out, and the old heating pad and aspirin just aren't cutting the mustard. Doc, I wouldn't complain, but I can barely get moving in the morning because my sleep is all jacked up. It hurts every time I roll over on that damn right hip. Hell, some mornings I just want to sit down and cry. Doc, can you just give me a quick shot or something to get me through calving season? You know as well as anybody if I don't get those calves to market, my kids and I don't eat."

I asked Addie about any antecedent trauma to the right hip. She thought about it for a minute and said that she got thrown from her horse onto her right hip when she was a teenager. She went on to say that Old Doc Jones "thought I just sprained my hip and I would be fine, and until the last few weeks when I was unloading bales of hay, he was right. He was a real crackerjack—Old Doc Jones. He delivered my mom and he delivered me. We put a lot of stock in what-ever Doc Jones told us and always did what he said."

I asked Addie to point with one finger to show me where it hurts the most. She pointed to the front of her right groin and said, "Doc, I got a hitch right here, especially when I first get up in the morning. The crazy thing is, sometimes I feel like the hip is popping or catching." I asked if she had any fever or chills and she shook her head no. "What about steroids? Did you ever take any cortisone or drugs like that?" Addie again shook her head no and said, "Doc, you know me. I am healthy as a horse. I love working the ranch, but this hitch has really got me down for the count." Addie denied any other gynecologic symptoms or blood in her urine.

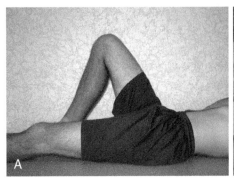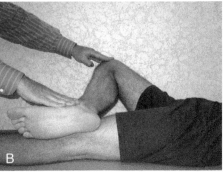

Fig. 1.1   Eliciting the Patrick (FABER) test. (From Waldman SD, *Physical Diagnosis of Pain: An Atlas of Signs and Symptoms*. 3rd ed. St Louis: Elsevier; 2016: Fig. 185-1.)

On physical examination, Addie was afebrile. Her respirations were 18 and her pulse was 74 and regular. Her blood pressure (BP) was normal at 122/74. Her head, eyes, ears, nose, throat (HEENT) exam was normal, as was her cardiopulmonary examination. Her thyroid was normal. Her abdominal examination revealed no abnormal mass or organomegaly. There was no costovertebral angle (CVA) tenderness. There was no peripheral edema. Her low back examination was unremarkable. I did a rectal exam and pelvic, which were both normal. Visual inspection of the right groin and hip revealed no cutaneous lesions or obvious hernia or other abnormal mass. The area overlying the right hip was cool to touch. Palpation of the right hip revealed mild diffuse tenderness, with no obvious effusion or point tenderness. There was mild crepitus, but I did not appreciate any popping or catching. Range of motion was decreased, with pain exacerbated with active and passive range of motion. When I performed the Patrick (FABER: flexion, abduction, external rotation) test on the right hip, Addie cried out in pain and said, "Doc, that's the hitch in my git-along!" (Fig. 1.1). The left hip examination was normal, as was examination of her other major joints, other than some mild osteoarthritis in the right hand. A careful neurologic examination of the upper and lower extremities revealed that there was no evidence of peripheral or entrapment neuropathy and the deep tendon reflexes were normal.

Key Clinical Points—What's Important and What's Not

THE HISTORY

- A distant history of acute trauma to the right hip secondary to falling from a horse
- No history of previous significant hip pain other than the short-term pain secondary to the acute hip trauma
- No fever or chills

- Gradual onset of right groin and hip pain over the last several weeks with exacerbation of pain with hip use
- Popping sensation in the right hip
- Sleep disturbance
- Difficulty walking secondary to pain upon first arising from the supine or recumbent position

THE PHYSICAL EXAMINATION

- The patient is afebrile
- Normal visual inspection of hip
- Palpation of right hip reveals diffuse tenderness
- No point tenderness
- No increased temperature of right hip
- Crepitus to palpation
- Positive Patrick (FABER) test on the right (see Fig. 1.1)

OTHER FINDINGS OF NOTE

- Normal BP
- Normal HEENT examination
- Normal cardiovascular examination
- Normal pulmonary examination
- Normal abdominal examination
- No peripheral edema
- No groin mass or inguinal hernia
- No CVA tenderness
- Normal pelvic exam
- Normal rectal exam
- Normal upper extremity neurologic examination, motor and sensory examination
- Examination of joints other than the right hip were normal

 What Tests Would You Like to Order?

The following tests were ordered:
- Plain radiographs of the right hip

TEST RESULTS

The plain radiographs of the right hip revealed significant joint space narrowing and osteophyte formation consistent with severe osteoarthritis (Fig. 1.2).

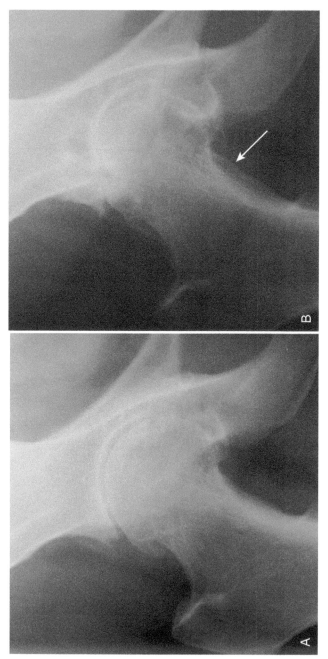

Fig. 1.2 (A) Anteroposterior (AP) radiograph of a patient with typical osteoarthritis (OA) of the hip with joint space narrowing and osteophyte formation. (B) A radiograph of the same patient acquired 18 months later shows rapid progression of the OA changes, with more marked superior joint space narrowing, supralateral migration of the femoral head, prominent subchondral cyst formation, and buttressing of the medial aspect of the femoral neck *(white arrow)*. (From Waldman SD, Campbell RSD. *Imaging of Pain.* Philadelphia: Saunders; 2011: Fig. 138-1.)

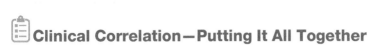

Clinical Correlation—Putting It All Together

What is the diagnosis?
- Osteoarthritis of the right hip joint

The Science Behind the Diagnosis

ANATOMY OF THE JOINTS OF THE HIP

The rounded head of the femur articulates with the cup-shaped acetabulum of the hip (Fig. 1.3). The articular surface is covered with hyaline cartilage, which is susceptible to arthritis. The rim of the acetabulum is composed of a fibrocartilaginous layer called the *acetabular labrum*, which is susceptible to trauma should the femur be subluxed or dislocated. The joint is surrounded by a capsule that allows the wide range of motion of the hip joint. The joint capsule is lined with a synovial membrane that attaches to the articular cartilage. This membrane gives rise to synovial tendon sheaths and bursae that are subject to inflammation. The hip joint is innervated by the femoral, obturator, and sciatic nerves. The major ligaments of the hip joint include the iliofemoral, pubofemoral, ischiofemoral, and transverse acetabular ligaments, which provide strength to the hip joint. The muscles of the hip and their attaching tendons are susceptible to trauma and to wear and tear from overuse and misuse.

CLINICAL PRESENTATION OF ARTHRITIS OF THE HIP JOINT

Most patients presenting with hip pain secondary to arthritis complain of pain localized around the hip and upper leg (Fig. 1.4). Most patients with intrinsic hip disorders have a positive Patrick (FABER) test result (see Fig. 1.1). Patients may initially present with ill-defined pain in the groin; occasionally, the pain is localized to the buttock. Activity makes the pain worse, whereas rest and heat provide some relief. The pain is constant and is characterized as aching; it may interfere with sleep. Some patients complain of a grating or popping sensation with use of the joint, and crepitus may be noted on physical examination.

In addition to pain, patients often experience a gradual decrease in functional ability caused by reduced hip range of motion that makes simple everyday tasks such as walking, climbing stairs, and getting into and out of a car quite difficult. With continued disuse, muscle wasting may occur, and a frozen hip secondary to adhesive capsulitis may develop.

TESTING

Plain radiography is indicated in all patients who present with hip pain. Based on the patient's clinical presentation, additional testing may be warranted,

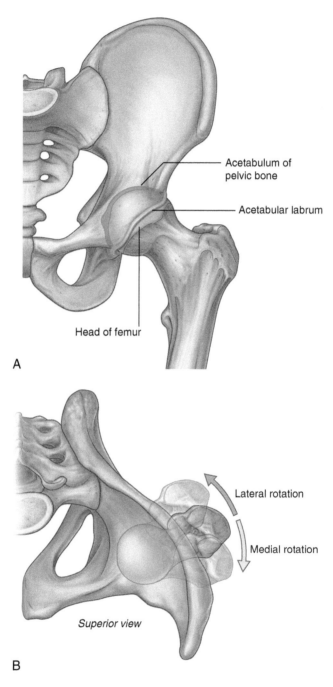

A

B

Fig. 1.3 The anatomy of the hip joint. (A) Articular surfaces. (B) Movement of the femur during rotation. (From Drake R, Vogl AW: *Gray's Anatomy for Students*. 4th ed. Philadelphia: Elsevier; 2020: Fig. 6-30.)

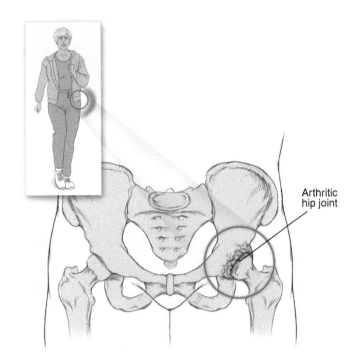

Fig. 1.4 Patients presenting with hip pain secondary to arthritis complain of pain localized around the hip and upper leg. (From Waldman SD. *Atlas of Common Pain Syndromes*. 4th ed. Philadelphia: Elsevier; 2019: Fig. 98-1.)

including a complete blood count, erythrocyte sedimentation rate, and antinuclear antibody testing. Magnetic resonance and ultrasound imaging of the hip are indicated if aseptic necrosis or an occult mass or tumor is suspected or if the diagnosis is in question (Figs. 1.5, 1.6, and 1.7).

DIFFERENTIAL DIAGNOSIS

Many diseases can cause hip pain (Table 1.1). Lumbar radiculopathy may mimic the pain and disability associated with arthritis of the hip; however, in such patients, hip examination results should be negative. Entrapment neuropathies, such as meralgia paresthetica, and trochanteric bursitis may confuse the diagnosis; both of these conditions can coexist with arthritis of the hip. Primary and metastatic tumors of the hip and spine may also manifest similarly to arthritis of the hip.

TREATMENT

Initial treatment of the pain and functional disability of arthritis of the hip includes a combination of nonsteroidal antiinflammatory drugs or

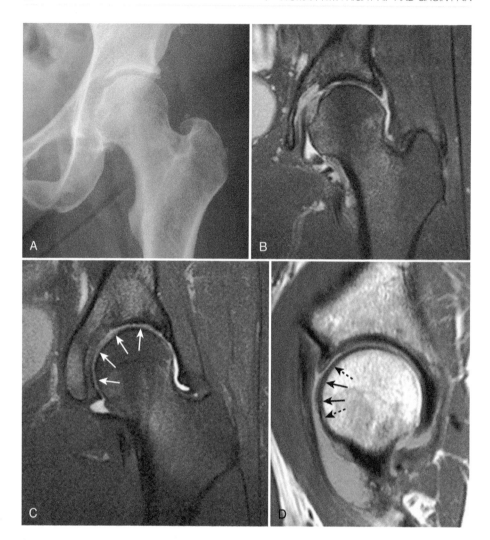

Fig. 1.5 (A) Anteroposterior (AP) radiograph of a 60-year-old patient with hip pain, which shows no significant osteoarthritis (OA) changes. (B) However, the coronal T2-weighted with fat suppression (FST2W) magnetic resonance (MR) image clearly demonstrates a high-signal intensity (SI) hip joint effusion with diffuse areas of cartilage loss across the femoral head due to early OA. (C) Compare with the FST2W MR image of a normal hip with intermediate-SI cartilage overlying the low-SI subchondral bone plate *(white arrows)*. (D) The cartilage loss is also seen on the sagittal proton density image *(broken black arrows)* but with some areas of cartilage preservation *(black arrows)*. (From Waldman SD, Campbell RSD. *Imaging of Pain*. Philadelphia: Saunders; 2011: Fig. 138-2.)

cyclooxygenase-2 inhibitors and physical therapy. The local application of heat and cold may also be beneficial. For patients who do not respond to these treatment modalities, intraarticular injection of local anesthetic and steroid is a reasonable next step.

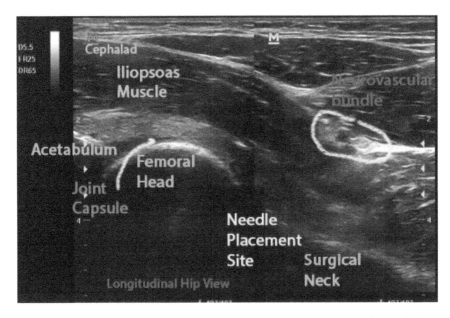

Fig. 1.6 Ultrasound image of the hip demonstrating the relationship of the acetabulum to the femoral head and joint capsule. (Courtesy Steven D. Waldman, MD.)

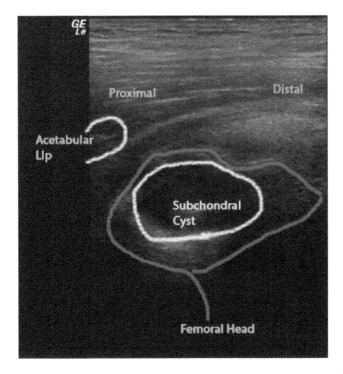

Fig. 1.7 Ultrasound image demonstrating avascular necrosis of the hip. (Courtesy Steven D. Waldman, MD.)

TABLE 1.1 ■ Causes of Hip Pain and Dysfunction

Localized Bony or Joint Space Pathology	Periarticular Pathology	Systemic Disease	Sympathetically Mediated Pain	Referred From Other Body Areas	Vascular Disease
Fracture	Bursitis	Rheumatoid arthritis	Causalgia	Lumbar plexopathy	Aortoiliac atherosclerosis
Primary bone tumor	Tendinitis	Collagen vascular disease	Reflex sympathetic dystrophy	Lumbar radiculopathy	Internal iliac artery occlusion
Primary synovial tissue tumor	Adhesive capsulitis	Reiter syndrome	Lumbar spondylosis	Entrapment neuropathies	
Joint instability	Joint instability	Gout	Fibromyalgia		
Localized arthritis	Muscle strain	Other crystal arthropathies	Myofascial pain syndromes		
Osteophyte formation	Muscle sprain	Charcot neuropathic arthritis	Inguinal hernia		
Osteonecrosis of femoral head	Periarticular infection not involving joint space				
Joint space infection					
Hemarthrosis					
Villonodular synovitis					
Intraarticular foreign body					
Slipped capital femoral epiphysis (Legg disease)					
Chronic hip dislocation					

From Waldman SD. *Atlas of Common Pain Syndromes*. 4th ed. Philadelphia: Elsevier; 2019: Table 98-1.

Intraarticular injection of the hip is performed by placing the patient in the supine position. The skin overlying the hip, subacromial region, and joint space is prepared with antiseptic solution. A sterile syringe containing 4 mL of 0.25% preservative-free bupivacaine and 40 mg methylprednisolone is attached to a 2-inch, 25-gauge needle by using strict aseptic technique. The femoral artery is identified; then, at a point approximately 2 inches lateral to the femoral artery, just below the inguinal ligament, the hip joint space is identified. The needle is carefully advanced through the skin and subcutaneous tissues through the joint capsule into the joint. If bone is encountered, the needle is withdrawn into the subcutaneous tissues and is redirected superiorly and slightly more medially. After the joint space is entered, the contents of the syringe are gently injected. Little resistance to injection should be felt. If resistance is encountered, the needle is probably in a ligament or tendon and should be advanced slightly into the joint space until the injection can proceed without significant resistance. The needle is removed, and a sterile pressure dressing and ice pack are applied to the injection site. Ultrasound needle guidance will simplify this procedure, improve the accuracy of needle placement, and decrease the incidence of needle-related complications (see Fig. 1.6). Recent clinical experience suggests that the intra- articular injection of platelet-rich plasma and/or stem cells may provide improvement of the pain and functional disability of patients suffering from osteroarthritis of the hip.

HIGH-YIELD TAKEAWAYS

- The patient is afebrile, making an acute infectious etiology (e.g., septic arthritis) unlikely.
- The patient's symptomatology is not the result of acute trauma but more likely the result of repetitive microtrauma that has damaged the joint over time.
- The patient's pain is diffuse rather than highly localized, as would be the case with a pathologic process like trochanteric bursitis.
- The patient's symptoms are unilateral and only involve one joint, which is more suggestive of a local process than a systemic polyarthropathy.
- Sleep disturbance is common and must be addressed concurrently with the patient's pain symptomatology.
- Plain radiographs will provide high-yield information regarding the bony contents of the joint, but ultrasound imaging and magnetic resonance imaging will be more useful in identifying soft tissue pathology.

Suggested Readings

Caughran AT, Giangarra CE. The arthritic hip. In: Giangarra CE, Manske RC, eds. *Clinical Orthopaedic Rehabilitation: A Team Approach*. 4th ed. Philadelphia: Elsevier; 2018:432−435.

El-Bakoury A, Williams M. Management of hip pain in young adults. *Surgery (Oxford)*. 2020;38(2):74–78.

Foye PM, Stitik TP, Shah VP, et al. Hip osteoarthritis. In: Frontera WR, Silver JK, Rizzo TD, eds. *Essentials of Physical Medicine and Rehabilitation*. 4th ed. Philadelphia: Elsevier; 2020:307–314.

Waldman SD. Arthritis and Other Abnormalities of the Hip Joint. In: *Waldman's Comprehensive Atlas of Diagnostic Ultrasound of Painful Conditions*. Philadelphia: Wolters Kluwer; 2016:613–622.

Arthritis pain of the hip. In: Waldman SD, ed. *Atlas of Common Pain Syndromes*. 4th ed. Philadelphia: Elsevier; 2019:383–386.

Waldman SD. *Hip Joint Pain Review*. 2nd ed. Philadelphia: Elsevier; 2017:140–141.

Waldman SD. Intra-articular injection of the hip. In: *Atlas of Pain Management Injection Techniques*. 4th ed. Philadelphia: Elsevier; 2017:385–390.

Waldman SD, Campbell RSD. Osteoarthritis of the Jip Joint. In: *Imaging of Pain*. Philadelphia: Saunders; 2011:351–352.

2

Sandy Brooks

A 69-Year-Old Female With Left Hip and Groin Pain

LEARNING OBJECTIVES

- Learn the common causes of hip pain.
- Develop an understanding of the unique anatomy of the hip joint.
- Develop an understanding of the causes of avascular necrosis of the hip.
- Learn the clinical presentation of avascular necrosis of the hip joint.
- Learn how to use physical examination to identify pathology of the hip joint.
- Develop an understanding of the treatment options for avascular necrosis of the hip joint.
- Learn the appropriate testing options to help diagnose avascular necrosis of the hip joint.
- Learn to identify red flags in patients who present with hip pain.
- Develop an understanding of the role in interventional pain management in the treatment of hip pain.

Sandy Brooks

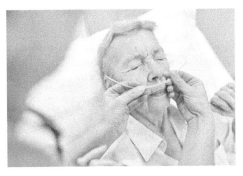

Sandy Brooks is a 69-year-old retired teacher with the chief complaint of, "My left hip hurts whenever I walk." She volunteered that her left hip had been bothering her for the last couple of years, but she hadn't realized how bad it had gotten because, until her pulmonologist upped her prednisone dose, her breathing had been so bad that she was primarily staying in her recliner all day long. "Doc, whatever you do, don't smoke those coffin nails! They did me in, and I don't want that to happen to you. Dealing with this oxygen 24 hours a day is no picnic." I reassured Sandy that I never smoked and had little intention of starting now, and she patted my hand and said, "Thank God!" I asked her, "Other than prednisone and breathing medicines, have you tried anything else to help the pain?" Sandy said she had "tried rubbing on the Australian Dream and took some Tylenol, but I guess the pain was just down too deep for them to work." Sandy also noted that she had to stop using her heating pad because she fell asleep with it on and she accidently burned herself. "Doc, I just don't have any strength anymore. I'll have you know that I was quite an athlete when I was younger. Now, it's all I can do to get up and go to the ladies' room."

I asked Sandy if she had ever injured her left hip before and she thought for a moment, and said, "You know, when I was 5 or 6 years old, I got hit by a car when I ran out into the street to get my ball and had a dislocated hip. I can't remember which one—it was so long ago. It's a wonder I remember my own name any more." I gave her shoulder a squeeze, smiled, and told her that she was doing great and that we were going to figure out what was wrong with that hip and do what we could to get it better.

I asked Sandy to point with one finger to show me where it hurt the most. She pointed to the front of her left groin and said, "Doc, it hurts way down deep, and it really gets my attention when I try to bear weight on it. I really dread having to get up to go to the ladies' room. It really hurts, but I don't want to have an accident." I asked, "Does the pain go anywhere?" and Sandy noted that sometimes it radiated to the side of her thigh. Sandy denied any gynecologic symptoms or blood in her urine.

On physical examination, Sandy was afebrile and dyspneic at rest. Her respirations were 22. Her pulse was 88 and regular. Her blood pressure (BP) was normal at 112/76. In spite of the recent increase in her prednisone dose, Sandy did not appear cushingoid, but she looked like she had lost a little weight since I had seen her for her flu shot. Her head, eyes, ears, nose, throat (HEENT) exam was normal, as was her thyroid examination. Her cardiopulmonary examination revealed diminished breath sounds with prolonged expiration and a few wheezes. Her abdominal examination revealed no abnormal mass or organomegaly. There was no costovertebral angle (CVA) tenderness. There was no peripheral edema. Her low back examination was unremarkable. I did a rectal and pelvic exam, which were both normal other than mild atrophic vaginitis. Visual inspection of the left groin and hip revealed no cutaneous lesions or obvious hernia or other abnormal mass. The area overlying the left hip was cool to touch. Palpation of the left hip revealed mild diffuse tenderness, with no obvious effusion or point tenderness. There was mild crepitus and I thought I detected a click with range of motion. The overall range of motion was decreased with pain exacerbated with active and passive range of motion. I had Sandy walk down the hall and noticed that she had a positive Hopalong Cassidy sign for antalgic gait (Fig. 2.1). The right hip examination was normal, as was examination of her other major joints, except for some mild osteoarthritis in the left hand. A careful neurologic examination of the upper and lower extremities revealed there was no

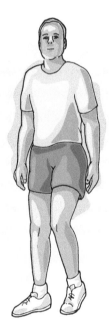

Fig. 2.1 The Hopalong Cassidy sign for antalgic gait. (From Waldman SD. *Physical Diagnosis of Pain: An Atlas of Signs and Symptoms*. 3rd ed. St Louis: Elsevier; 2016: Fig. 184-3.)

evidence of peripheral or entrapment neuropathy, and the deep tendon reflexes were normal.

Key Clinical Points—What's Important and What's Not

THE HISTORY

- A history of a recent increase in prednisone dose to treat an exacerbation of chronic obstructive pulmonary disease (COPD)
- A questionable distant history of acute trauma to the left hip/dislocation after being hit by a car
- A several-year history of some left hip pain with a recent acute exacerbation after an increase in prednisone dosage
- Increase in pain with weight bearing
- No fever or chills

THE PHYSICAL EXAMINATION

- The patient is afebrile
- Normal visual inspection of hip
- Palpation of left hip reveals diffuse tenderness
- No point tenderness
- No increased temperature of left hip
- Crepitus to palpation during range of motion of left hip
- Click sensation during range of motion of left hip
- Positive Hopalong Cassidy sign on the left (see Fig. 2.1)

OTHER FINDINGS OF NOTE

- Normal BP
- Normal HEENT examination
- Normal cardiovascular examination
- Abnormal pulmonary examination
- Normal abdominal examination
- No peripheral edema
- No groin mass or inguinal hernia
- No CVA tenderness
- Normal pelvic exam
- Normal rectal exam
- Normal upper extremity neurologic examination, motor and sensory examination
- Examinations of joints other than the left hip were normal

What Tests Would You Like to Order?

The following tests were ordered:
- Plain radiograph of the left hip
- Magnetic resonance imaging (MRI) of the left hip

Test Results

The plain radiographs of the left hip revealed sclerotic changes of the femoral head consistent with advanced avascular necrosis (Figs. 2.2 and 2.3).

 Clinical Correlation—Putting It All Together

What is the diagnosis?
- Avascular necrosis (osteonecrosis) of the left hip joint

The Science Behind the Diagnosis

ANATOMY OF THE HIP JOINTS

The rounded head of the femur articulates with the cup-shaped acetabulum of the hip. The articular surface is covered with hyaline cartilage, which is

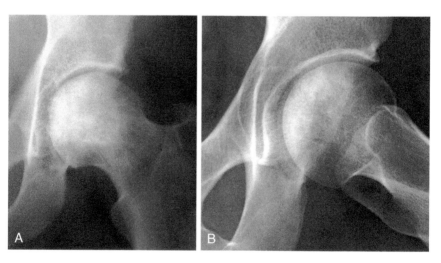

Fig. 2.2 Anteroposterior (A) and frog-leg (B) views of the left hip showing sclerotic changes of the femoral head typical of advanced osteonecrosis. (From Firestein G, et al. *Kelley and Firestein's Textbook of Rheumatology.* 10th ed. Philadelphia: Elsevier; 2017: Fig. 103-4.)

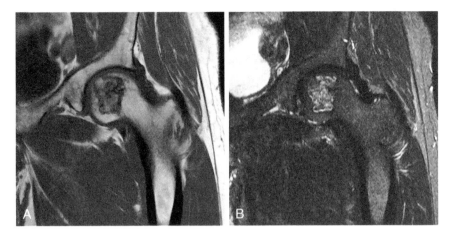

Fig. 2.3 Magnetic resonance imaging (MRI) of the left hip. (A) T1-weighted coronal MRI of the left hip revealed an osteonecrotic segment in the subchondral portion of the femoral head with low signal intensity. (B) T2-weighted coronal MRI revealed the necrotic bone, which exhibited high signal intensity, surrounded by a sclerotic low signal rim. (From Firestein GS, Budd RC, Gabriel SE, *Kelley and Firestein's Textbook of Rheumatology*. 10th ed. Philadelphia: Elsevier; 2017 [Fig. 103-8].)

susceptible to arthritis. The rim of the acetabulum is composed of a fibrocartilaginous layer called the acetabular labrum, which is susceptible to trauma should the femur be subluxed or dislocated. The joint is surrounded by a capsule that allows the wide range of motion of the hip joint. The joint capsule is lined with a synovial membrane that attaches to the articular cartilage. This membrane gives rise to synovial tendon sheaths and bursae that are subject to inflammation. The hip joint is innervated by the femoral, obturator, and sciatic nerves. The blood supply to the femoral head is variable, but some generalizations can be made. Branches arising from the deep femoral artery give rise to the superior, inferior, anterior, and posterior retinacular arteries. Additional blood supply to the femoral head arises from the artery of the ligamentum teres, which is a branch of the obturator artery (Fig. 2.4). This blood supply is easily disrupted by trauma. The major ligaments of the hip joint include the iliofemoral, pubofemoral, ischiofemoral, and transverse acetabular ligaments, which provide strength to the hip joint. The muscles of the hip and their attaching tendons are susceptible to trauma and to wear and tear from overuse and misuse.

CLINICAL PRESENTATION OF AVASCULAR NECROSIS OF THE HIP JOINT

Avascular necrosis of the hip is an often missed diagnosis. It is also known as osteonecrosis. Similar to the scaphoid, the hip is extremely susceptible to this

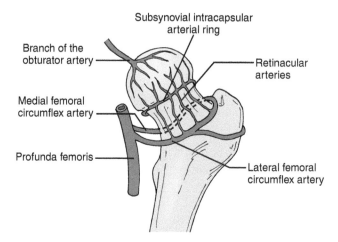

Fig. 2.4   The blood supply of the femoral head. (From Firestein GS, Budd RC, Gabriel SE, *Kelley and Firestein's Textbook of Rheumatology.* 10th ed. Philadelphia: Elsevier; 2017: Fig. 103-1.)

disease because of its tenuous blood supply. The blood supply of the hip is easily disrupted, often leaving the proximal portion of the bone without nutrition, thereby leading to osteonecrosis. Avascular necrosis of the hip is a disease of the fourth and fifth decades of life and is more common in men, with an 8:1 male-to-female preponderance (Fig. 2.5), except for patients with avascular necrosis of the hip secondary to collagen vascular disease. The disease is bilateral in 50% to 55% of cases.

Predisposing factors to avascular necrosis of the hip are listed in Table 2.1 and include trauma to the proximal femur and acetabulum, corticosteroid use, Cushing disease, alcohol abuse, connective tissue diseases (especially systemic lupus erythematous), osteomyelitis, human immunodeficiency virus (HIV), organ transplantation, Legg-Calvé-Perthes disease, hemoglobinopathies (including sickle cell disease), hyperlipidemia, gout, renal failure, pregnancy, and radiation therapy involving the femoral head. A patient with avascular necrosis of the hip reports pain over the affected hip(s), which may radiate into the groin, buttock, and proximal lower extremity. The pain is deep and aching, and the patient often reports a catching sensation with range of motion of the affected hip(s). Range of motion decreases as the disease progresses.

Physical examination of patients with avascular necrosis of the hip reveals pain to deep palpation of the hip joint. The pain becomes worse with passive range of motion and weight bearing on a single extremity. A click or crepitus may be appreciated by the examiner when putting the hip joint through range of motion. A Trendelenburg or antalgic gait with its characteristic Hopalong Cassidy sign may be noted, and decreased range of motion is invariably present (see Fig. 2.1).

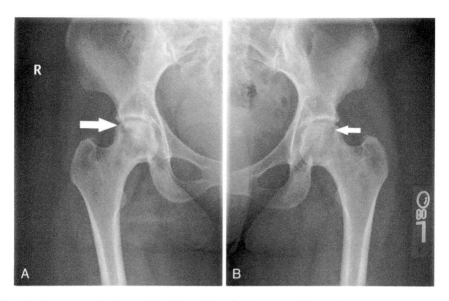

Fig. 2.5 Anteroposterior views of the bilateral hips. Radiographs of the patient's right (A) and left (B) hips both demonstrate femoral head sclerotic changes with subchondral lucency consistent with crescent sign (*arrows*) and femoral head collapse consistent with Steinberg stage IV osteonecrosis (bilateral hip avascular necrosis). (From April M, Watts R, Hunter C. Avascular necrosis of the hip. *J Emerg Med*. 2015;49(4):e115—e116 [Fig. 1].)

TABLE 2.1 ■ **Predisposing Factors for Avascular Necrosis of the Hip**

Trauma to proximal femur and acetabulum
Corticosteroid use
Cushing disease
Alcohol abuse
Connective tissue diseases, especially systemic lupus erythematosus
Osteomyelitis
Human immunodeficiency virus
Organ transplantation
Legg-Calvé-Perthes disease
Hemoglobinopathies, including sickle cell disease
Hyperlipidemia
Gout
Renal failure
Pregnancy
Radiation therapy

TESTING

Plain radiographs are indicated in all patients with avascular necrosis of the hip to rule out underlying occult bony pathologic processes and identify sclerosis and fragmentation of the femoral head, although early in the course of the disease, plain radiographs are unreliable (see Fig. 2.2). Based on the patient's clinical presentation, additional tests, including complete blood cell count, uric acid, erythrocyte sedimentation rate, and antinuclear antibody testing, may be indicated. MRI of the hip is indicated in all patients suspected to have avascular necrosis of the hip or if other causes of joint instability, infection, or tumor are suspected (Fig. 2.6; see Fig. 2.3). Administration of gadolinium followed by

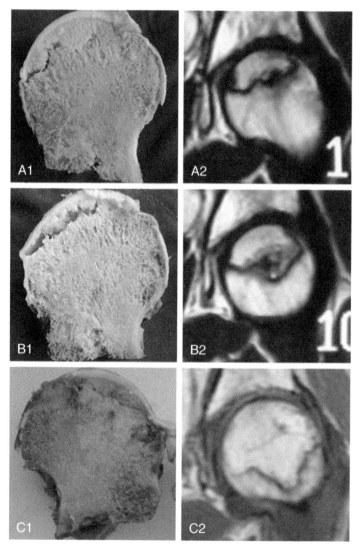

Fig 2.6   Gross specimens of femoral head osteonecrosis (A1, B1, C1) and the relative magnetic resonance images. (A2, B2, C2) (From Chen L, Hong GJ, Fang B, et al. Predicting the collapse of the femoral head due to osteonecrosis: from basic methods to application prospects. *J Orthop Trans*. 2017;11:62–72 [Fig. 1].)

postcontrast imaging may help delineate the adequacy of blood supply, with contrast enhancement of the proximal hip being a good prognostic sign. Computed tomography scanning and ultrasound imaging may provide additional information regarding the condition of the hip joint and guide treatment decisions (Figs. 2.7 and 2.8). Electromyography is indicated if coexistent lumbar radiculopathy, plexopathy, or both are suspected. A gentle injection of the hip joint with small volumes of local anesthetic provides immediate improvement of the pain and helps show the nidus of the patient's pain is, in fact, the hip. Ultimately, total joint replacement is required in most patients with avascular necrosis of the hip.

DIFFERENTIAL DIAGNOSIS

Coexistent arthritis, crystal deposition diseases, and gout of the hip joints, bursitis, and tendinitis may coexist with avascular necrosis of the hips and exacerbate the pain and disability of the patient (Fig. 2.9). Tears of the labrum, ligament tears, bone cysts, bone contusions, bone fractures, and occult metastatic disease also may mimic the pain of avascular necrosis of the hip.

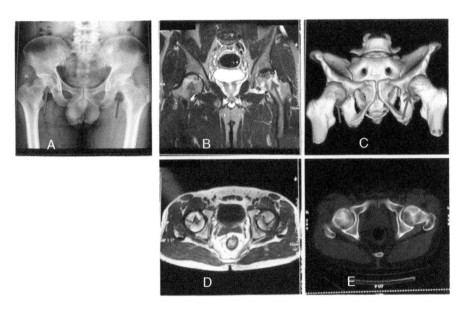

Fig 2.7 (A) Dual X-ray absorptiometry, (B) magnetic resonance imaging (MRI), and (C) computed tomography (CT) of a 41-year-old man with bilateral osteonecrosis of the femoral head *(red arrows)*, and showing the Ficat and Arlet stage II and III lesions in the right and left femoral heads, respectively. The volume, angle, and arc of osteonecrotic lesions are detected on (D) MRI and (E) CT for guiding further treatment. (From Cao H, Guan H, Lai Y, et al. Review of various treatment options and potential therapies for osteonecrosis of the femoral head. *J Orthop Trans*. 2016;4:57–70 [Fig. 1].)

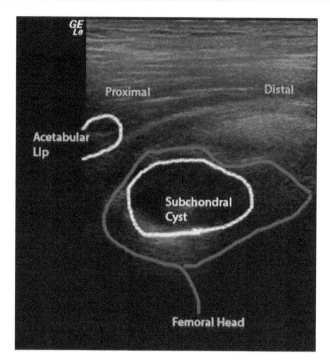

Fig. 2.8 Ultrasound image demonstrating avascular necrosis of the hip. (Courtesy Steven D. Waldman, MD.)

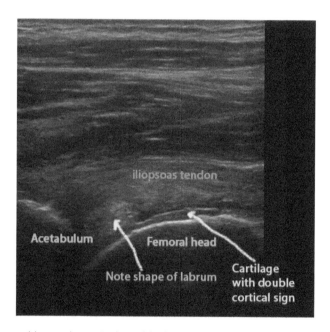

Fig. 2.9 Ultrasound image demonstrating a labral tear in a patient with gout. (Courtesy Steven D. Waldman, MD.)

TREATMENT

Initial treatment of the pain and functional disability associated with avascular necrosis of the hip should include a combination of nonsteroidal antiinflammatory drugs or cyclooxygenase-2 inhibitors and decreased weight bearing of the affected hip(s). Local application of heat and cold may be beneficial. For patients who do not respond to these treatment modalities, an injection of a local anesthetic into the hip joint may be a reasonable next step to provide palliation of acute pain. Vigorous exercises should be avoided because they would exacerbate the patient's symptoms. Ultimately, surgical repair in the form of total joint arthroplasty is the treatment of choice.

HIGH-YIELD TAKEAWAYS

- The patient is afebrile, making an acute infectious etiology (e.g., septic arthritis) unlikely.
- The patient's symptomatology is not the result of acute trauma, although the history of hip dislocation should suggest the potential for avascular necrosis.
- The patient's pain is diffuse rather than highly localized as would be the case with a pathologic process such as trochanteric bursitis.
- The patient's symptoms are unilateral and involve only one joint, which is more suggestive of a local process than a systemic polyarthropathy.
- Sleep disturbance is common and must be addressed concurrently with the patient's pain symptomatology.
- Pain on ambulation in the elderly is an important risk factor, and assistive devices such as a quad-cane or walker may help mitigate the risk of falling.
- Plain radiographs will provide high-yield information regarding the bony contents of the joint, but ultrasound imaging and MRI will be more useful in identifying soft tissue pathology.

Suggested Readings

Chen L, Hong G, Fang B, et al. Predicting the collapse of the femoral head due to osteonecrosis: from basic methods to application prospects. *J Orthop Trans*. 2017;11: 62—72.

El-Bakoury A, Williams M. Management of hip pain in young adults. *Surgery (Oxford)*. 2020;38(2):74—78.

Kubo T, Ueshima K, Saito M, et al. Clinical and basic research on steroid-induced osteonecrosis of the femoral head in Japan. *J Orthop Sci*. 2016;21(4):407—413.

Saito M, Ueshima K, Ishida M, et al. Alcohol-associated osteonecrosis of the femoral head with subsequent development in the contralateral hip: a report of two cases. *J Orthop Sci*. 2016;21(6):870—874.

Waldman SD. Arthritis and Other Abnormalities of the Hip Joint. In: *Waldman's Comprehensive Atlas of Diagnostic Ultrasound of Painful Conditions*. Philadelphia: Wolters Kluwer; 2016:613–622.

Waldman SD. Hip Joint. In: *Pain Review*. 2nd ed. Philadelphia: Elsevier; 2017:140–141.

Waldman SD. Intra-articular Injection of the Hip. In: *Atlas of Pain Management Injection Techniques*. 4th ed. Philadelphia: Elsevier; 2017:385–390.

Waldman SD, Campbell RSD. Osteonecrosis of the Hip. In: *Imaging of Pain*. Philadelphia: Saunders; 2011:339–342.

Beth Nash

A 25-Year-Old Female With Right Groin Pain

- Learn the common causes of groin pain.
- Develop an understanding of the anatomy of the nerves of the lumbosacral plexus.
- Develop an understanding of the causes of ilioinguinal neuralgia.
- Learn the clinical presentation of ilioinguinal neuralgia.
- Learn how to use physical examination to identify ilioinguinal neuralgia.
- Develop an understanding of the treatment options for ilioinguinal neuralgia.
- Learn the appropriate testing options to help diagnose ilioinguinal neuralgia.
- Learn to identify red flags in patients who present with groin pain.
- Develop an understanding of the role of interventional pain management in the treatment of ilioinguinal neuralgia.

Beth Nash

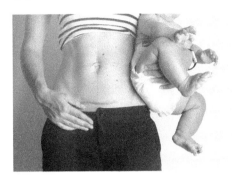

Beth Nash is a 25-year-old respiratory therapist with the chief complaint of, "I've got a shooting pain into my groin since my C-section." Beth went on to say that "other than the shooting pain, Buster and I have been doing great since our C-section." I assumed that Buster was the rambunctious 6-month-old who was trying to escape his mother's grasp. I asked Beth if this was her first child and she smiled brightly and said, "Yes, he is, and he is a real handful! Doctor, it's been great except for this pain. At first I thought it was just postsurgical pain, but as I healed up, this shooting pain into my groin just wouldn't go away. The crazy thing is, I feel like I can't stand up straight, because when I do, I get this electric shock into my privates. Bill, my husband, says I am walking around like an old lady!"

I asked Beth if she ever had anything like this before, and she shook her head no. She also denied any other urinary or gynecologic symptoms, hematuria, or fever or chills. She also denied a history of kidney stones. She had started her periods again with her last menstrual period a week ago. Beth was using condoms for birth control, as she was still breast feeding. I asked what she was doing to manage the pain and she said that "nothing really works." I asked her to rate her pain on a scale of 1 to 10, with 10 being the worst pain she had ever had, and she said the shocks were a 7 or 8. "Doctor, if I have to live with the pain, I can, but it is interfering with everything—getting dressed, taking care of Buster, sex—everything. I just never know when it's going to hit." Beth said that she looked up post-C-section pain on the Internet, and she wasn't trying to be the doctor, but as best as she could tell, she thought it might be nerve damage from the incision. She gave me an inquisitive look, and I smiled and said that I thought that she was spot on. "Let's take a look at you and see if we both have the correct diagnosis."

I asked my nurse to hold Buster, then asked Beth to point with one finger to show me where it hurt the most. She pointed to the front of her right groin and said, "Doc, the pain shoots down into my right labia. The C-section incision itself doesn't hurt, but there is this spot just below the incision that if I push on it, bang! It causes the electric shock—it really gets my attention. I'm worried it will hit and I will drop Buster."

On physical examination, Beth was afebrile. Her respirations were 16. Her pulse was 68 and regular. Her blood pressure (BP) was normal at 110/70. Her nutrition appeared fine. Her head, eyes, ears, nose, and throat (HEENT) exam was normal, as was her thyroid examination. Her cardiopulmonary examination was negative. Her abdominal examination revealed no abnormal mass or organomegaly. There was no costovertebral angle (CVA) tenderness. There was no peripheral edema. Her low back examination was unremarkable. Her lower extremity neurologic examination was completely normal.

I asked Beth to lie back on the examination table with her knees bent so we could take a closer look at her cesarean section scar. Visual inspection of the scar revealed no obvious defect or infection. Inspection of the groin revealed no obvious abnormal mass or inguinal hernia. I again asked Beth to use one finger to point to the spot that caused the shooting pain, and she carefully pointed to a spot about 2 inches medial to the anterior superior iliac spine and 2 inches below that spot (Fig. 3.1). This spot was just below the lateral aspect of the cesarean section scar. I asked Beth if I could palpate the spot that she identified and, after a moment's hesitation, she nodded yes and said, "Sure, just be gentle." I said, "No problem. Why don't you

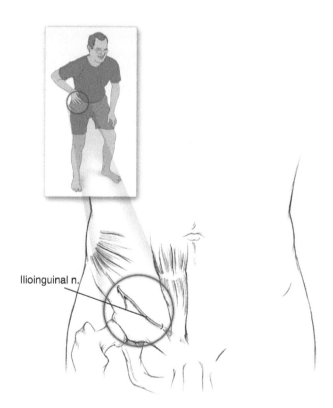

Ilioinguinal n.

Fig. 3.1 The location of the ilioinguinal nerve in relation to the anterior superior iliac spine. (From Waldman SD. *Atlas of Common Pain Syndromes*. 4th ed. Philadelphia: Elsevier; 2019: Fig. 80.1.)

hold my hand, and you do the pushing and I'll do the feeling so together we'll figure out what is going on." She liked that idea, so I had Beth guide my index finger to the spot that was causing the trouble. There was no obvious surgical defect, but there was allodynia, and when Beth tentatively pushed my index finger into the spot just below the scar, I felt her suddenly withdraw her pelvis as she said, "Right there!" I said, "I think we have our answer. How about getting up and walking down the hall for me?" She carefully sat up and slid off the exam table, immediately assuming the novice skier position (Fig. 3.2). When I asked her to stand up straight, the pain recurred and she reassumed the novice skier position.

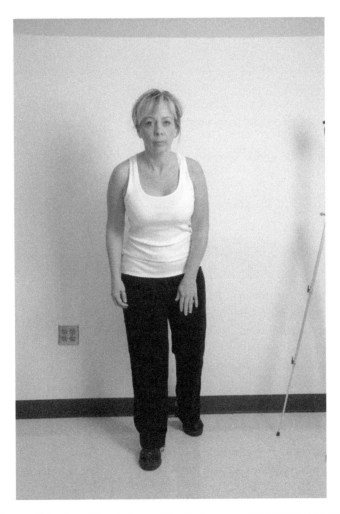

Fig. 3.2   Patients suffering from ilioinguinal neuralgia will often assume the novice skier position.

Key Clinical Points—What's Important and What's Not

THE HISTORY

- A history of recent onset right-sided groin pain following a cesarean section
- No history of urinary or gynecologic symptoms related to the pain
- No history of kidney stones
- No history of hematuria
- Difficulty in assuming the full upright position without eliciting pain
- Pain has an electric shocklike quality
- A spot just below the lateral aspect of the cesarean section scar that elicits pain on palpation
- No fever or chills

THE PHYSICAL EXAMINATION

- The patient is afebrile
- Normal visual inspection of the cesarean section scar
- Palpation of a discrete point approximately 2 inches medial to the anterior superior iliac spine and 2 inches below that spot elicits a shocklike pain into the right labia
- Patient assumes novice skier position when walking
- Pain is elicited when patient is asked to assume full upright position (Fig. 3.3)
- The lower extremity neurologic examination is within normal limits

OTHER FINDINGS OF NOTE

- Normal BP
- Normal HEENT examination
- Normal cardiopulmonary examination
- Normal abdominal examination
- No peripheral edema
- No groin mass or inguinal hernia
- No CVA tenderness

 ## What Tests Would You Like to Order?

The following tests were ordered:

- Electromyography (EMG) and nerve conduction studies of the ilioinguinal, iliohypogastric, and genitofemoral nerves
- Ultrasound imaging of the ilioinguinal, iliohypogastric, and genitofemoral nerves and surrounding area

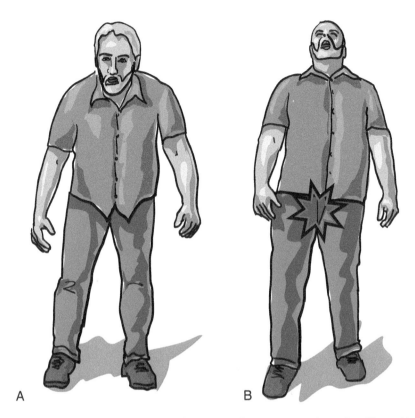

A   B

Fig. 3.3 (A) Patients suffering from ilioinguinal neuralgia will often assume the novice skier position to relieve pressure or tension on the affected ilioinguinal nerve. (B) Pain is often elicited when the patient is asked to assume the full upright position. (From Waldman SD. *Physical Diagnosis of Pain: An Atlas of Signs and Symptoms*. 3rd ed. St Louis: Elsevier; 2016: Fig. 169-1.)

TEST RESULTS

The EMG and nerve conduction studies of the ilioinguinal, iliohypogastric, and genitofemoral nerves revealed mild denervation of the internal oblique muscle on the right and slowing of the nerve conduction of the ilioinguinal nerve on the right. The remainder of the examination was within normal limits (Table 3.1). Ultrasound imaging of the ilioinguinal, iliohypogastric, and genitofemoral nerves and surrounding area revealed no abnormal mass compressing the ilioinguinal or iliohypogastric nerve or obvious neuroma of the ilioinguinal nerve (Fig. 3.4).

Clinical Correlation—Putting It All Together

What is the diagnosis?
- Ilioinguinal neuralgia

TABLE 3.1 ■ Distribution of the Ilioinguinal, Iliohypogastric, and Genitofemoral Nerves

Nerve	Nerve Roots	Cutaneous Innervation	Motor Innervation
Iliohypogastric	T12–L1	Lower abdomen Superior mons pubis Lateral gluteal	Internal oblique
Ilioinguinal	T12–L1	Superomedial thigh Base of penis Anterior scrotum Labium majora Mons pubis	Internal oblique
Genitofemoral	L1–L2	Superior anterior thigh Scrotum Labia	Cremaster

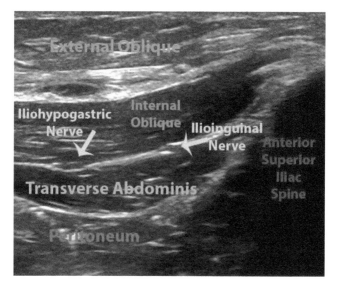

Fig. 3.4 Ultrasound imaging of the ilioinguinal and iliohypogastric nerves. Note the relationship of the ilioinguinal nerve to the anterior superior iliac spine. (Courtesy Steven D. Waldman.)

The Science Behind the Diagnosis

ANATOMY OF THE ILIOINGUINAL NERVE

The ilioinguinal nerve is derived from the L1 nerve root with a contribution from T12 in some patients. The nerve exits the lateral border of the psoas muscle to follow a curvilinear course that takes it from its origin of the L1 and occasionally T12 somatic nerves to inside the concavity of the ilium (Fig. 3.5). The ilioinguinal nerve continues in an anterior trajectory as it runs between the layers of the

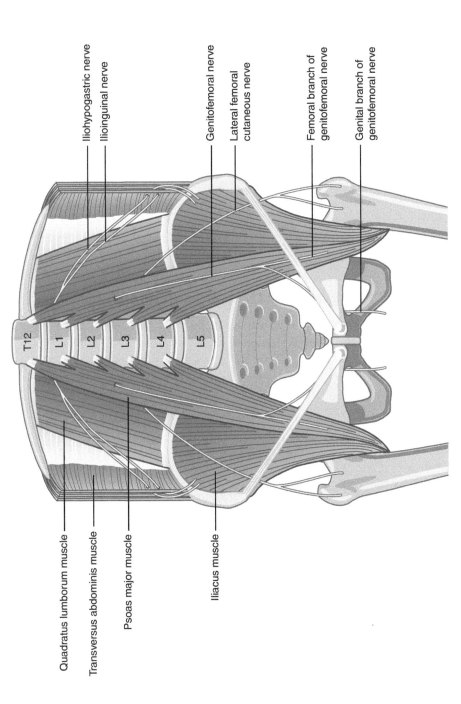

Iliohypogastric nerve

Ilioinguinal nerve

Genitofemoral nerve

Lateral femoral cutaneous nerve

Femoral branch of genitofemoral nerve

Genital branch of genitofemoral nerve

Quadratus lumborum muscle

Transversus abdominis muscle

Psoas major muscle

Iliacus muscle

T12

L1

L2

L3

L4

L5

Fig. 3.5 Course of the ilioinguinal, iliohypogastric, and genitofemoral nerves as they leave the lumbar plexus and pass through the muscular layers of the abdomen. (From Waldman SD. *Atlas of Interventional Pain Management.* 4th ed. Philadelphia: Saunders; 2015: Fig. 86.3.)

internal oblique and transversus abdominis muscles. It is at this point that the nerve can consistently be identified with ultrasound scanning and is amenable to ultrasound-guided nerve block. The ilioinguinal nerve then perforates the transverse abdominis muscle at the level of the anterior superior iliac spine, and its terminal branches provide sensory innervation to the skin over the inferior portion of the rectus abdominis muscle. The ilioinguinal nerve may interconnect with the iliohypogastric nerve as it continues to pass along its course medially and inferiorly, where it accompanies the genital branch of the genitofemoral nerve as well as the spermatic cord in men and the round ligament in women through the inguinal ring and into the inguinal canal. The distribution of the sensory innervation of the ilioinguinal nerves varies from patient to patient due to considerable overlap with the iliohypogastric nerve. In most patients, the ilioinguinal nerve provides sensory innervation to the upper portion of the skin of the inner thigh and the root of the penis and upper scrotum in men or the mons pubis and lateral labia in women (Fig. 3.6).

CLINICAL PRESENTATION OF ILIOINGUINAL NEURALGIA

Ilioinguinal neuralgia presents as paresthesias, burning pain, and occasionally numbness over the lower abdomen that radiates into the scrotum or labia and occasionally into the upper inner thigh; pain does not radiate below the knee. The pain of ilioinguinal neuralgia is made worse by extension of the lumbar spine, which puts traction on the nerve; thus patients often assume a bent-forward, novice skier's position (see Fig. 3.3). If the condition remains untreated, progressive motor deficit, consisting of bulging of the anterior abdominal wall muscles, may occur. This bulging may be confused with inguinal hernia.

Physical findings include sensory deficit in the inner thigh, scrotum, or labia in the distribution of the ilioinguinal nerve. Weakness of the anterior abdominal wall musculature may be present. Tinel sign may be elicited by tapping over the ilioinguinal nerve at the point where it pierces the transverse abdominal muscle.

TESTING

EMG can distinguish ilioinguinal nerve entrapment from lumbar plexopathy, lumbar radiculopathy, and diabetic polyneuropathy. Plain radiographs of the hip and pelvis are indicated in all patients who present with ilioinguinal neuralgia to rule out occult bony pathology. Based on the patient's clinical presentation, additional testing may be warranted, including a complete blood count, uric acid level, erythrocyte sedimentation rate, and antinuclear antibody testing.

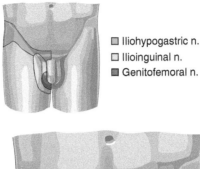

☐ Iliohypogastric n.
☐ Ilioinguinal n.
■ Genitofemoral n.

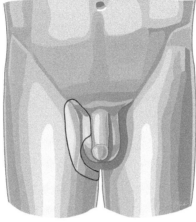

☐ Ilioinguinal n.

Fig. 3.6 The distribution of the sensory innervation of the ilioinguinal nerves varies from patient to patient due to considerable overlap with the iliohypogastric nerve. In most patients, the ilioinguinal nerve provides sensory innervation to the upper portion of the skin of the inner thigh and the root of the penis and upper scrotum in men or the mons pubis and lateral labia in women. (From Waldman SD. *Atlas of Interventional Pain Management*. 4th ed. Philadelphia: Saunders; 2015: Fig. 86.5.)

Ultrasound imaging of the ilioinguinal nerve may aid in the identification of masses or tumors compressing the ilioinguinal nerve or posttraumatic neuromas of the nerve (see Fig. 3.4). Magnetic resonance imaging (MRI) of the lumbar plexus is indicated if tumor or hematoma is suspected (Fig. 3.7). The injection technique described later serves as both a diagnostic and a therapeutic maneuver.

DIFFERENTIAL DIAGNOSIS

Lesions of the lumbar plexus caused by trauma, hematoma, tumor, diabetic neuropathy, or inflammation can mimic the pain, numbness, and weakness of ilioinguinal neuralgia and must be ruled out (see Fig. 3.7). Further, there is significant variability in the anatomy of the ilioinguinal nerve, which can result in significant variation in the clinical presentation.

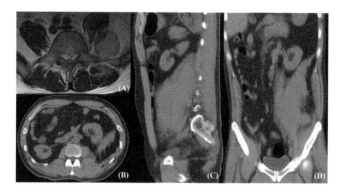

Fig. 3.7 Axial magnetic resonance imaging shows an anterior shift of the left psoas muscle caused by the retroperitoneal hematoma (A, C). At 7 h after surgery, the change of the hematoma to a diffuse type was confirmed on coronal abdominal computed tomography images (B, D). The volume was measured to be 810 mL (20 cm × 9 cm × 9 cm × 0.5), and the hematoma was pushing the left kidney in a superior and ventral direction. (From Bae D-H, Eun S-S, Lee S-H, et al. Two cases of retroperitoneal hematoma after transforaminal percutaneous endoscopic lumbar discectomy. *Interdiscipl Neurosurg.* 2020:20:100649 [Fig. 2].)

TREATMENT

Initial treatment of ilioinguinal neuralgia consists of simple analgesics, nonsteroidal antiinflammatory drugs, or cyclooxygenase-2 inhibitors. Avoidance of repetitive activities thought to exacerbate the pain (e.g., squatting or sitting for prolonged periods) may also ameliorate the patient's symptoms. Pharmacologic treatment is usually disappointing, however, in which case ilioinguinal nerve block with local anesthetic and steroid is required.

Ilioinguinal nerve block is performed with the patient in the supine position; a pillow can be placed under the patient's knees if lying with the legs extended increases the pain due to traction on the nerve. The anterior superior iliac spine is identified by palpation, and a point 2 inches medial and 2 inches inferior to it is identified and prepared with antiseptic solution. A 1.5-inch, 25-gauge needle is advanced at an oblique angle toward the pubic symphysis (Fig. 3.8). A total of 5 to 7 mL of 1% preservative-free lidocaine in solution with 40 mg methylprednisolone is injected in a fanlike manner as the needle pierces the fascia of the external oblique muscle. Care must be taken not to insert the needle too deeply, which risks entering the peritoneal cavity and perforating the abdominal viscera. Because of the overlapping innervation of the ilioinguinal and iliohypogastric nerves, it is usually not necessary to block branches of each nerve. After injection of the solution, pressure is applied to the injection site to decrease the incidence of ecchymosis and hematoma formation, which can be quite dramatic, especially in anticoagulated patients. If anatomic landmarks are unclear, the use of fluoroscopic or ultrasound guidance should be considered (see Fig. 3.4).

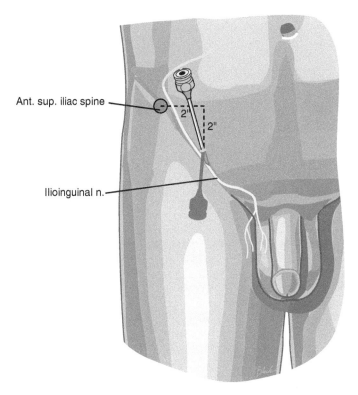

Ant. sup. iliac spine

2"   2"

Ilioinguinal n.

Fig. 3.8 At a point 2 inches medial and 2 inches inferior to the anterior superior iliac spine, a 1.5-inch, 25-gauge needle is inserted through the skin and advanced at an oblique angle toward the pubic symphysis to place the needle tip in proximity to the ilioinguinal nerve. (From Waldman SD. *Atlas of Interventional Pain Management*. 4th ed. Philadelphia: Saunders; 2015: Fig. 86.6.)

For patients who do not rapidly respond to ilioinguinal nerve block, consideration should be given to epidural steroid injection of the T12–L1 segments.

HIGH-YIELD TAKEAWAYS

- The patient's symptomatology began after a surgical procedure in the region of the ilioinguinal nerve.
- The patient is afebrile, making an acute infectious etiology (e.g., postoperative infection or urosepsis) unlikely.
- The lower extremity neurologic examination is within normal limits, making a central spinal or lumbar plexus lesion much less likely.
- The character of the pain is shocklike, suggesting a neurogenic etiology.

(Continued)

- The EMG and nerve conduction were abnormal, suggesting a localized lesion, with clinical correlation specifically pointing toward a diagnosis of ilioinguinal neuralgia.
- If a lesion of the spinal cord or lumbar plexus is being considered, MRI of the lumbar spine and lumbar plexus is indicated.
- Ultrasound imaging will be helpful in identifying local pathology compromising the ilioingional nerve as well as discrete lesions of the ilioinguinal nerve (e.g., neuroma).

Suggested Readings

Bhatia N, Sen IM, Mandal B, et al. Postoperative analgesic efficacy of ultrasound-guided ilioinguinal-iliohypogastric nerve block compared with medial transverse abdominis plane block in inguinal hernia repair: a prospective, randomised trial. *Anaesth Crit Care Pain Med.* 2019;38(1):41–45.

Waldman SD. Iliohypogastric Nerve Entrapment. In: *Waldman's Comprehensive Atlas of Diagnostic Ultrasound of Painful Conditions.* Philadelphia: Wolters Kluwer; 2016:587–595.

Waldman SD. Ilioinguinal Nerve Block. In: *Pain Review.* 2nd ed. Philadelphia: Saunders; 2017:474–476.

Waldman SD. Ilioinguinal Nerve Entrapment. In: *Waldman's Comprehensive Atlas of Diagnostic Ultrasound of Painful Conditions.* Philadelphia: Wolters Kluwer; 2016:580–587.

Waldman SD. Ilioinguinal Neuralgia. In: *Atlas of Common Pain Syndromes.* 4th ed. Philadelphia: Elsevier; 2017:311–314.

Waldman SD. Orchalgia. In: *Atlas of Uncommon Pain Syndromes.* 3rd ed. Philadelphia: Saunders; 2014:251–254.

Bob Hamilton

A 42-Year-Old Male With Numbness in the Lateral Thigh

- Learn the common causes of lower extremity numbness.
- Develop an understanding of the unique relationship of the lateral femoral cutaneous nerve to the inguinal ligaments.
- Develop an understanding of the anatomy of the lateral femoral cutaneous nerve.
- Develop an understanding of the causes of meralgia paresthetica.
- Develop an understanding of the differential diagnosis of meralgia paresthetica.
- Learn the clinical presentation of meralgia paresthetica.
- Learn the dermatomes of the lower extremity.
- Learn how to use physical examination to identify meralgia paresthetica.
- Develop an understanding of the treatment options for meralgia paresthetica.

Bob Hamilton

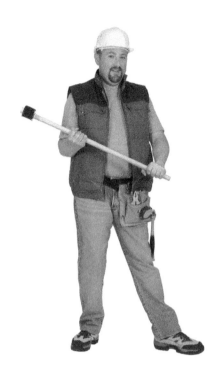

Bob Hamilton is a 42-year-old construction worker with the chief complaint of, "I have burning pain and numbness in the side of my left thigh." Bob stated that over the past several months, he began noticing that he started getting a pins-and-needles sensation in his left thigh after he had been sitting in his recliner watching Netflix. He noted that if he didn't get up and move around that the sensation would get worse until he just had to get up to "shake it off." I asked Bob if he had experienced any numbness or weakness in his legs and he replied, "Doc, it's funny that you asked, because over the last couple of weeks, if I am squatting down at work for any length of time, my left leg gets continually more numb." "Both legs?" I asked, and he said no, only the left leg. "Bob, does this pins-and-needles sensation and numbness go below the knee?" He shook his head and said, "Never." (Fig. 4.1) I asked Bob what he thought was causing his symptoms and after a moment he replied, "Doc, this may be crazy, but I am beginning to wonder if it is my tool belt." I asked Bob what he had tried to make it better and he said that he had tried shifting his tool belt to the right side, but it made it harder to get his tools out, and taking Motrin just upset his stomach. He said that he also tried not putting the leg rest all the way up on his recliner to take pressure off his bum leg. He also volunteered that he had quit sleeping with his pajama bottoms because the skin over the numb area was so sensitive. "It's kinda like a burn. Also, Tylenol PM seems to help some—at least with sleep." "Interesting," I said. "Any intentional weight loss or weight gain?" Bob gave me a sheepish grin and said, "I know, Doc, I need to cut back on the beer and Doritos. I have really packed it on since my leg started bothering me."

I asked Bob to show me where the pins-and-needles sensation and numbness were and he pointed to his left lateral thigh. "Right here, Doc, and it's really driving me crazy." I asked Bob about any fever, chills, or other constitutional symptoms such as weight loss, night sweats, etc., and

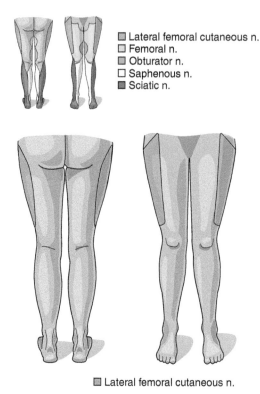

☐ Lateral femoral cutaneous n.
☐ Femoral n.
☐ Obturator n.
☐ Saphenous n.
■ Sciatic n.

☐ Lateral femoral cutaneous n.

Fig. 4.1 The sensory distribution of the lateral femoral cutaneous nerve. *n*, nerve. (From Waldman SD. *Atlas of Interventional Pain Management*. 4th ed. Philadelphia: Saunders; 2015: Fig. 125-4.)

he just shook his head no. He denied any antecedent lower extremity trauma, but noted that sometimes the pins-and-needles pain woke him up at night.

He went on to say that he could live with the numbness, but the pins-and-needles pain and the sensitive skin were really bothering him. He then asked, "Doc, do you think this could be cancer? You know, my dad died of colon cancer last year, and this really has me freaked out." I clapped Bob on the shoulder and said that I was pretty sure what was causing his symptoms, and I seriously doubted it was cancer.

On physical examination, Bob was afebrile. His respirations were 18, his pulse was 74 and regular, and his blood pressure (BP) was 132/78. His body mass index (BMI) was 35.2. His head, eyes, ears, nose, throat (HEENT) exam was normal, as was his cardiopulmonary examination. His thyroid was normal. His abdominal examination revealed no abnormal mass or organomegaly. There was no costovertebral angle (CVA) tenderness. There was no peripheral edema. His low back examination was unremarkable. Visual inspection of the left lower extremity was unremarkable. There was no rubor or color, but there was allodynia in the distribution of the lateral femoral cutaneous nerve on the left. There was no obvious infection. I asked Bob to squat; after about 30 seconds he had to stand up because the pins-and-needles sensation was too much for him to tolerate.

A careful neurologic examination of both lower extremities revealed decreased sensation in the distribution of the left lateral femoral cutaneous nerve, but no sensory abnormalities below the knee were identified (Fig. 4.2). His left motor exam was within normal limits. His right lower extremity neurologic examination was completely normal. Deep tendon reflexes were normal bilaterally. There was a positive Tinel sign over the left lateral femoral cutaneous nerve (Fig. 4.3).

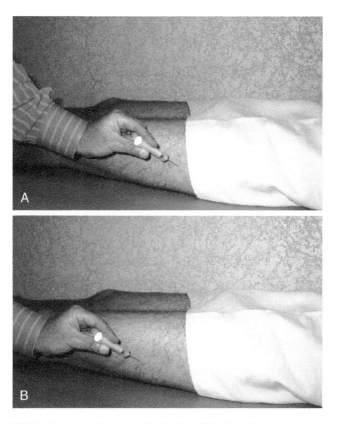

Fig. 4.2 (A and B) Checking sensation in the distribution of the lateral femoral cutaneous nerve. (From Waldman SD. *Physical Diagnosis of Pain: An Atlas of Signs and Symptoms*. 3rd ed. St Louis: Elsevier; 2016: Fig. 171-2A,B.)

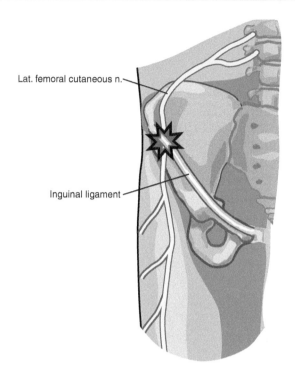

Fig. 4.3 Location of Tinel test of the lateral femoral cutaneous nerve at the level of the inguinal liga-ment. *n*, nerve. (From Waldman SD. *Physical Diagnosis of Pain: An Atlas of Signs and Symptoms.* 3rd ed. St Louis: Elsevier; 2016: Fig. 171-1.)

Key Clinical Points—What's Important and What's Not

THE HISTORY

- A history of onset of a pins-and-needles sensation of the left lateral thigh that does not radiate below the knee
- Numbness of the left lateral thigh that does not radiate below the knee
- Pins-and-needles sensation and numbness exacerbated by sitting or squatting for long periods of time
- No symptoms in the right lower extremity
- History of recent weight gain
- History of wearing a heavy tool belt
- No fever or chills

THE PHYSICAL EXAMINATION

- The patient is afebrile
- High BMI

- Positive Tinel sign over the lateral femoral cutaneous nerve on the left (see Fig. 4.3)
- Decreased sensation in the distribution of the left lateral femoral cutaneous nerve
- Allodynia in the distribution of the left lateral femoral cutaneous nerve
- No motor deficit in the right lower extremity
- Deep tendon reflexes within normal limits bilaterally

OTHER FINDINGS OF NOTE

- Normal HEENT examination
- Normal cardiovascular examination
- Normal pulmonary examination
- Normal abdominal examination
- No peripheral edema

 ## What Tests Would You Like to Order?

The following tests were ordered:
- Ultrasound of the left lateral femoral cutaneous nerve at the level of the inguinal ligament
- Electromyography (EMG) and nerve conduction velocity testing of the left lateral femoral cutaneous nerve

TEST RESULTS

Ultrasound examination of the lateral femoral cutaneous nerve at the level of the femoral triangle reveals no obvious tumor or mass compressing the lateral femoral cutaneous nerve (Fig. 4.4). EMG and nerve conduction velocity testing revealed slowing of lateral femoral cutaneous nerve conduction across the femoral triangle.

 ## Clinical Correlation—Putting It All Together

What is the diagnosis?
- Meralgia paresthetica

The Science Behind the Diagnosis
ANATOMY

The lateral femoral cutaneous nerve is formed from the posterior divisions of the L2 and L3 nerves of the lumbar plexus (Fig. 4.5). The nerve leaves the psoas

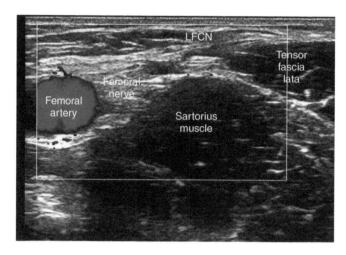

Fig. 4.4 Ultrasound imaging of the lateral femoral cutaneous nerve *(LFCN)* at the level of the femoral triangle. (From Waldman SD. *Atlas of Interventional Pain Management*. 4th ed. Philadelphia: Saunders; 2015: Fig. 125-10.)

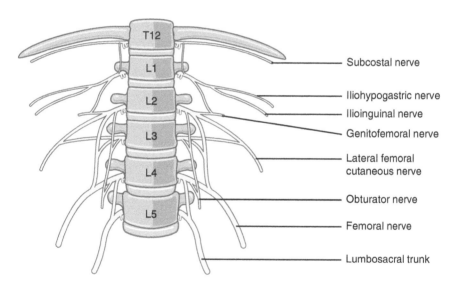

Fig. 4.5 The lateral femoral cutaneous nerve is formed from the posterior divisions of the L2 and L3 nerves of the lumbar plexus. (From Waldman SD. *Atlas of Interventional Pain Management*. 4th ed. Philadelphia: Saunders; 2015: Fig. 125-2.)

muscle and courses laterally and inferiorly to pass just beneath the ilioinguinal nerve at the level of the anterior-superior iliac spine (Fig. 4.6). The nerve passes under the inguinal ligament and then travels beneath the fascia lata, where it divides into an anterior and a posterior branch. The anterior branch provides limited cutaneous sensory innervation over the anterolateral thigh. The posterior

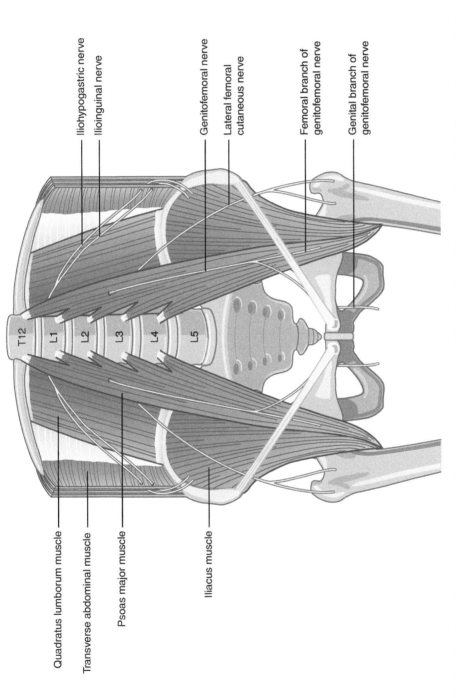

Iliohypogastric nerve

Ilioinguinal nerve

Genitofemoral nerve

Lateral femoral
cutaneous nerve

Femoral branch of
genitofemoral nerve

Genital branch of
genitofemoral nerve

T12

L1

L2

L3

L4

L5

Quadratus lumborum muscle

Transverse abdominal muscle

Psoas major muscle

Iliacus muscle

Fig. 4.6 The lateral femoral cutaneous nerve leaves the psoas muscle and courses laterally and inferiorly to pass just beneath the ilioinguinal nerve at the level of the anterior-superior iliac spine. The nerve passes under the inguinal ligament and then travels beneath the fascia lata, where it divides into an anterior and a posterior branch. (From Waldman SD. *Atlas of Interventional Pain Management*. 4th ed. Philadelphia: Saunders; 2015: Fig. 125-3.)

branch provides cutaneous sensory innervation to the lateral thigh from just above the greater trochanter to the knee (see Fig. 4.1).

CLINICAL SYNDROME

Meralgia paresthetica is caused by compression of the lateral femoral cutaneous nerve by the inguinal ligament. This entrapment neuropathy presents as pain, numbness, and dysesthesias in the distribution of the lateral femoral cutaneous nerve. The symptoms often begin as a burning pain in the lateral thigh, with associated cutaneous sensitivity. Patients suffering from meralgia paresthetica note that sitting, squatting, or wearing wide belts causes the symptoms to worsen (Fig. 4.7). Although traumatic lesions to the lateral femoral cutaneous nerve have been implicated in meralgia paresthetica, in most patients, no obvious antecedent trauma can be identified.

SIGNS AND SYMPTOMS

Physical findings include tenderness over the lateral femoral cutaneous nerve at the origin of the inguinal ligament at the anterior superior iliac spine. A positive Tinel sign over the lateral femoral cutaneous nerve as it passes beneath the inguinal ligament may be present. Patients may complain of burning dysesthesias in the nerve's distribution (see Fig. 4.1). Careful sensory examination of the lateral thigh reveals a sensory deficit in the distribution of the lateral femoral cutaneous nerve; no motor deficit should be present (see Fig. 4.2). Sitting or the wearing of tight waistbands or wide belts can compress the nerve and exacerbate the symptoms of meralgia paresthetica.

TESTING

Electromyography can distinguish lumbar radiculopathy and diabetic femoral neuropathy from meralgia paresthetica. Plain radiographs of the back, hip, and pelvis are indicated in selected patients who present with meralgia paresthetica to rule out occult bony pathology. Based on the patient's clinical presentation, additional testing may be warranted, including a complete blood count, uric acid level, erythrocyte sedimentation rate, and antinuclear antibody testing. Magnetic resonance imaging (MRI) of the back and lumbar plexus is indicated if herniated disk, spinal stenosis, or space-occupying lesion is suspected. Ultrasound imaging of the lateral femoral cutaneous nerve may be helpful in identifying tumors and masses compressing the nerve as well as tumors of the nerve itself (see Fig. 4.4). Injection of the lateral femoral cutaneous nerve with local anesthetic may serve as both a diagnostic and a therapeutic maneuver (Fig. 4.8).

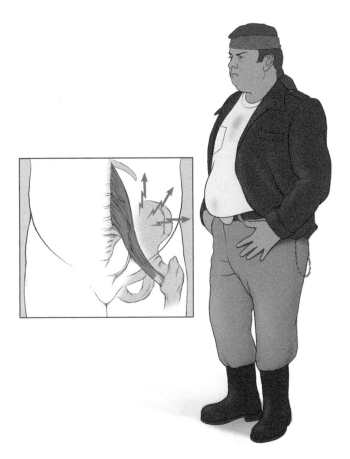

Fig. 4.7 Meralgia paresthetica is caused by compression of the lateral femoral cutaneous nerve by the inguinal ligament. This entrapment neuropathy presents as pain, numbness, and dysesthesias in the distribution of the lateral femoral cutaneous nerve. The symptoms often begin as a burning pain in the lateral thigh, with associated cutaneous sensitivity. Patients suffering from meralgia paresthetica note that sitting, squatting, or wearing wide belts causes the symptoms to worsen. (From Waldman SD. *Atlas of Interventional Pain Management*. 4th ed. Philadelphia: Saunders; 2015: Fig. 125-1.)

DIFFERENTIAL DIAGNOSIS

Meralgia paresthetica is often misdiagnosed as lumbar radiculopathy, trochanteric bursitis, or primary hip pathology. Radiographs of the hip and EMG can distinguish meralgia paresthetica from radiculopathy or pain emanating from the hip. In addition, most patients suffering from lumbar radiculopathy have back pain associated with reflex, motor, and sensory changes, whereas patients with meralgia paresthetica have no back pain and no motor or reflex changes; the sensory changes of meralgia paresthetica are limited to the distribution of the lateral femoral cutaneous nerve and should not extend below the knee. It should

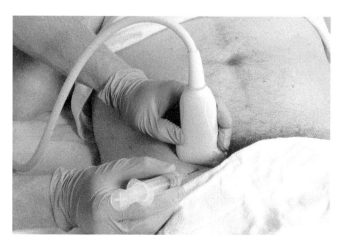

Fig. 4.8 Ultrasound-guided injection of the lateral femoral cutaneous nerve with local anesthetic may serve as both a diagnostic and a therapeutic maneuver. (From Waldman SD. *Atlas of Interventional Pain Management*. 4th ed. Philadelphia: Saunders; 2015: Fig. 125-11.)

be remembered that lumbar radiculopathy and lateral femoral cutaneous nerve entrapment may coexist as the "double crush" syndrome. Occasionally, diabetic femoral neuropathy produces anterior thigh pain, which may confuse the diagnosis.

TREATMENT

Patients suffering from meralgia paresthetica should be instructed in avoidance techniques to reduce the symptoms and pain associated with this entrapment neuropathy. A short course of conservative therapy consisting of simple analgesics, nonsteroidal antiinflammatory drugs, or cyclooxygenase-2 inhibitors is a reasonable first step in the treatment of meralgia paresthetica. If patients do not experience rapid improvement, injection of the lateral femoral cutaneous nerve with local anesthetic and/or steroid at the level of entrapment is the next step (see Fig. 4.8).

HIGH-YIELD TAKEAWAYS

- The patient is afebrile, making an acute infectious etiology unlikely.
- The patient's symptomatology is thought to be the result of compression of the left lateral femoral cutaneous nerve by a heavy tool belt.
- The patient may be predisposed to the development of meralgia paresthetica because of his obesity.

(Continued)

- Physical examination and testing should be focused on the identification of the other pathologic processes that may mimic the clinical diagnosis of meralgia paresthetica.
- The patient exhibits the neurologic and physical examination findings that are highly suggestive of meralgia paresthetica.
- The patient's pain does not go below the knee, which mitigates against radiculopathy or a more central spinal process.
- The patient's symptoms are unilateral.
- EMG and nerve conduction velocity testing will help delineate the location and degree of nerve compromise if lateral femoral cutaneous nerve compression is suspected.
- Ultrasound imaging of the lateral femoral cutaneous nerve may help identify less common causes of compression of the nerve (e.g., tumor, lipoma, or neural tumors).

Suggested Readings

Dimitropoulos G, Schaepkens van Riempst J, Schertenleib P. Anatomical variation of the lateral femoral cutaneous nerve: a case report and review of the literature. *J Plastic Reconstr Aesthet Surg.* 2011;64(7):961–962.

Lee B, Stubbs E. Sartorius muscle tear presenting as acute meralgia paresthetica. *Clin Imaging.* 2018;51:209–212.

Moucharafieh R, Wehbe J, Maalouf G. Meralgia paresthetica: a result of tight new trendy low cut trousers ('taille basse'). *Int J Surg.* 2008;6(2):164–168.

Waldman SD. Abnormalities of the Lateral Cutaneous Nerve. In: *Comprehensive Atlas of Diagnosis Ultrasound of Painful Conditions.* Philadelphia: Wolters Kluwer; 2016: 629–634.

Waldman SD. Meralgia Paresthetica. In: *Atlas of Common Pain Syndromes.* 4th ed. Philadelphia: Elsevier; 2019:399–402.

Becky Hanna

A 27-Year-Old Female With Severe Left Hip Pain

- Learn the common causes of hip pain.
- Develop an understanding of the unique anatomy of the hip joint.
- Develop an understanding of the bursae of the hip.
- Develop an understanding of the causes of trochanteric bursitis.
- Develop an understanding of the differential diagnosis of trochanteric bursitis.
- Learn the clinical presentation of trochanteric bursitis.
- Learn how to examine the hip and associated bursae.
- Learn how to use physical examination to identify trochanteric bursitis.
- Develop an understanding of the treatment options for trochanteric bursitis.

Becky Hanna

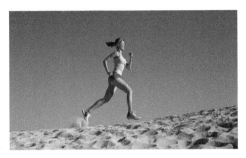

Becky Hanna is a 27-year-old sales representative with the chief complaint of, "My left hip is killing me." Becky stated that she was traveling to a sales meeting in Hilton Head about 3 weeks ago when she developed left hip pain after jogging on the beach. "Doctor, I am really fit. I had on pretty good shoes. I jog every day, but I'm not used to running on sand. I knew better than to run on sand, but the beach was just so beautiful—but I knew better." I told her not to be too hard on herself, that we would figure out what was going on.

I asked Becky about any antecedent hip trauma and she just shook her head no, but went on to say that from time to time, her left hip would bother her a little after completing a marathon, but a couple of Advil and she was good to go. This time, the pain just wouldn't go away in spite of using the Advil and a heating pad. Becky said the side of her hip was somewhat swollen and "squishy," and that it felt hot to touch. I asked Becky what made her pain worse and she said, "Any time I start to walk or run, I feel a sudden, sharp pain and a kind of catching sensation. Doctor, my hip really hurts and the pain is messing with my sleep. Every time I roll over onto my left side, the pain in my left hip wakes me up."

I asked Becky to point with one finger to show me where it hurt the most. She pointed to a spot just over the greater trochanter on the left and said, "Doctor, it hurts right here!"

On physical examination, Becky was afebrile. Her respirations were 18 and her pulse was 64 and regular. Her blood pressure was 118/68. Becky's head, eyes, ears, nose, and throat (HEENT) exam was normal, as was her cardiopulmonary examination. Her thyroid was normal. Her abdominal examination revealed no abnormal mass or organomegaly. There was no costovertebral angle (CVA) tenderness. There was no peripheral edema. Her low back examination was unremarkable. Visual inspection of the left lateral hip revealed mild swelling. The area over the left greater trochanter was warm but did not appear to be infected. The left hip felt "boggy" on palpation, and there was marked point tenderness over the greater trochanter. Palpation of the left greater trochanter area exacerbated Becky's pain. Range of motion of the hip joint, especially resisted abduction of the joint, caused Becky to cry out in pain. I performed a resisted abduction release

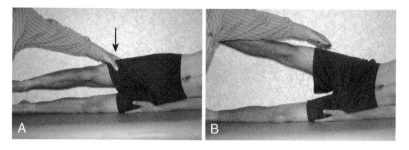

Fig. 5.1 (A, B) The resisted abduction release test for trochanteric bursitis. (From Waldman SD. *Physical Diagnosis of Pain: An Atlas of Signs and Symptoms*. 3rd ed. St Louis: Elsevier; 2016: Fig. 191-2 A,B.)

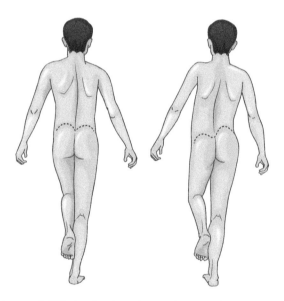

Fig. 5.2 Trendelenburg gait. With functional weakness of the hip abductor muscles, it is difficult to support the body's weight on the affected side; the pelvis tilts down and away from the weak side, the patient leans toward the affected side. (From Kleigman R, Lye PS, Bordini B, et al. *Nelson Pediatric Symptom-Based Diagnosis*. Gait disturbance by Shayne D. Fehr, Philadelphia: Elsevier; 2018.)

test, which was markedly positive on the left and negative on the right (Fig. 5.1). The right hip examination was normal, as was examination of her other major joints. A careful neurologic examination of the upper and lower extremities revealed there was no evidence of peripheral or entrapment neuropathy, and the deep tendon reflexes were normal. I asked Becky to walk down the hall, where I noted a Trendelenburg gait was present (Fig. 5.2).

Key Clinical Points—What's Important and What's Not

THE HISTORY

- Acute onset of left hip pain following running on a soft, sandy surface
- Pain localized to the area of the left greater trochanter
- Pain associated with a catching sensation
- No other specific traumatic event to the area identified
- History of mild self-limited left hip pain after running marathons
- No fever or chills
- Sleep disturbance
- Difficulty walking or running

THE PHYSICAL EXAMINATION

- The patient is afebrile
- Point tenderness to palpation of the area over the trochanteric bursa
- Palpation of left hip reveals warmth to touch
- The left lateral hip is swollen with "bogginess" over the left greater trochanter
- No evidence of infection
- Pain on range of motion, especially resisted abduction of the affected left hip
- The resisted abduction release test was positive on the left (see Fig. 5.1)
- A Trendelenburg gait was present (see Fig. 5.2)

OTHER FINDINGS OF NOTE

- Normal HEENT examination
- Normal cardiovascular examination
- Normal pulmonary examination
- Normal abdominal examination
- No peripheral edema
- Normal upper and lower extremity neurologic examination, motor and sensory examination
- Examinations of other joints other than the left hip were normal

 ## What Tests Would You Like to Order?

The following tests were ordered:
- Plain radiographs of the left hip
- Ultrasound of the left hip

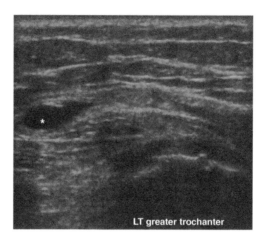

LT greater trochanter

Fig. 5.3 Longitudinal ultrasound image of trochanteric bursitis. Note the fluid collection within the bursa *(asterisk)*. (From Waldman SD. *Atlas of Pain Management Injection Techniques*. 4th ed. St Louis: Elsevier; 2017: Fig. 116-4.)

TEST RESULTS

The plain radiographs of the left hip were reported as normal. Specifically, there was no calcification in the area of the trochanteric bursa suggestive of chronic bursitis. Ultrasound examination of the left hip revealed an effusion around the trochanteric bursa (Fig. 5.3).

Clinical Correlation—Putting It All Together

What is the diagnosis?
- Trochanteric bursitis

The Science Behind the Diagnosis

ANATOMY

The trochanteric bursa lies between the greater trochanter and the tendon of the gluteus medius and the iliotibial tract. The gluteus medius muscle has its origin from the outer surface of the ilium, and its fibers pass downward and laterally to attach on the lateral surface of the greater trochanter. The gluteus medius locks the pelvis in place when walking and running. This action can irritate the trochanteric bursa, as can repeated trauma from repetitive activity, including jogging on soft or uneven surfaces or overuse of exercise equipment for lower extremity strengthening. The gluteus medius muscle is innervated by the superior gluteal nerve.

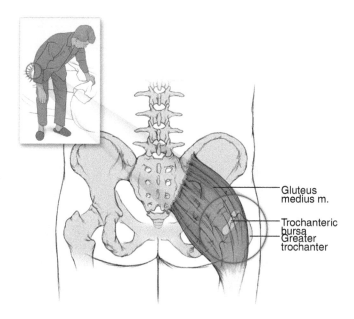

Fig. 5.4 The pain of trochanteric bursitis often mimics that of sciatica. *m*, muscle. (From Waldman SD. *Atlas of Common Pain Syndromes*. 4th ed. Philadelphia: Elsevier; 2019: Fig. 104.1.)

CLINICAL SYNDROME

Trochanteric bursitis is commonly encountered in clinical practice. Patients suffering from trochanteric bursitis frequently complain of pain in the lateral hip that occasionally radiates down the leg, mimicking sciatica (Fig. 5.4). The pain is localized to the area over the trochanter. Often, patients are unable to sleep on the affected hip and may complain of a sharp "catching" sensation with range of motion of the hip, especially on first arising. Patients may note that walking upstairs is becoming increasingly difficult. Trochanteric bursitis often coexists with arthritis of the hip and back, sacroiliac joint disease, and gait disturbance.

The trochanteric bursa lies between the greater trochanter and the tendon of the gluteus medius and the iliotibial tract (Fig. 5.5). This bursa may exist as a single bursal sac or, in some patients, as a multisegmented series of loculated sacs. The trochanteric bursa is vulnerable to injury from both acute trauma and repeated microtrauma. Acute injuries may be caused by direct trauma to the bursa from falls onto the greater trochanter or previous hip surgery, as well as by overuse injuries, including running on soft or uneven surfaces. If inflammation of the trochanteric bursa becomes chronic, calcification may occur.

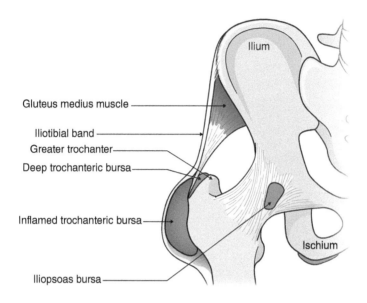

Fig. 5.5 The trochanteric bursa lies between the greater trochanter and the tendon of the gluteus medius and the iliotibial tract. This bursa may exist as a single bursal sac or, in some patients, as a multisegmented series of loculated sacs.

SIGNS AND SYMPTOMS

Physical examination reveals point tenderness in the lateral thigh just over the greater trochanter. Passive adduction and abduction, as well as active resisted abduction, of the affected lower extremity reproduce the pain. Sudden release of resistance during this maneuver causes a marked increase in pain (see Fig. 5.1). There should be no sensory deficit in the distribution of the lateral femoral cutaneous nerve; this distinguishes trochanteric bursitis from meralgia paresthetica. A Trendelenburg gait may be present as the patient tries to splint the inflamed area (see Fig. 5.2).

TESTING

Plain radiographs of the hip may reveal calcification of the bursa and associated structures, consistent with chronic inflammation (Fig. 5.6). Magnetic resonance imaging (MRI) is indicated if occult mass or tumor of the hip or groin is suspected or to confirm the diagnosis (Fig. 5.7). A complete blood count and erythrocyte sedimentation rate are useful if infection is suspected. Electromyography (EMG) can distinguish trochanteric bursitis from meralgia paresthetica and sciatica. Injection of the trochanteric bursa with local anesthetic and steroid may serve as both a diagnostic and a therapeutic maneuver (Fig. 5.8).

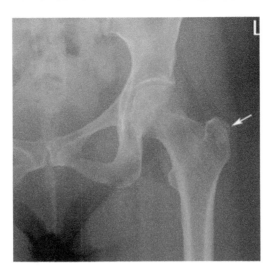

Fig 5.6 Plain radiograph demonstrating calcification *(arrow)* superficial to the greater trochanter consistent with calcific trochanteric bursitis and/or tendinitis. (From Mallow M, Nazarian LN. Greater trochanteric pain syndrome diagnosis and treatment. *Phys Med Rehab Clin North Am.* 2014;25 (2):279–289 [Fig. 6].)

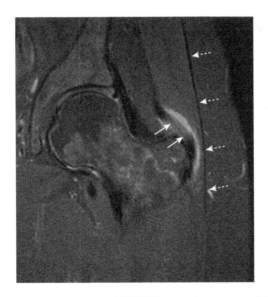

Fig. 5.7 Coronal fat suppressed T-2 weighted (FST2W) magnetic resonance (MR) image of a patient with lateral hip pain and trochanteric bursitis with high signal intensity fluid lying between the iliotibial tract *(broken white arrows)* and the gluteus minimus tendon *(white arrows)*. (From Waldman SD, Campbell RSD. *Imaging of Pain.* Philadelphia: Saunders; 2011: Fig. 142.2.)

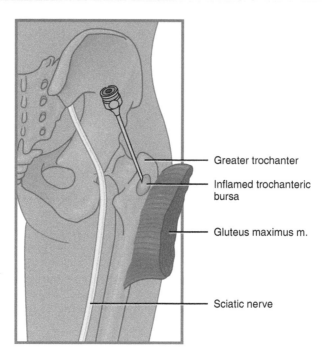

Greater trochanter

Inflamed trochanteric
bursa

Gluteus maximus m.

Sciatic nerve

Fig. 5.8 Injection of the trochanteric bursa with local anesthetic and steroid may serve as both a diagnostic and a therapeutic maneuver. *m*, muscles. (From Waldman SD. *Atlas of Pain Management Injection Techniques*. 4th ed. St Louis: Elsevier; 2017: Fig. 116-6.)

DIFFERENTIAL DIAGNOSIS

Trochanteric bursitis frequently coexists with arthritis of the hip. Occasionally, trochanteric bursitis can be confused with meralgia paresthetica because both present with pain in the lateral thigh; however, in patients with meralgia paresthetica, palpation over the greater trochanter does not elicit pain. EMG can help sort out confusing clinical presentations. Primary or secondary tumors of the hip must also be considered in the differential diagnosis of trochanteric bursitis. Other conditions that are associated with lateral hip pain that may mimic trochanteric bursitis are listed in Table 5.1.

TREATMENT

A short course of conservative therapy consisting of simple analgesics, nonsteroidal antiinflammatory drugs (NSAIDs), or cyclooxygenase-2 inhibitors is a reasonable first step in the treatment of trochanteric bursitis. Patients should be instructed to avoid repetitive activities that may be responsible for the development of trochanteric bursitis, such as running on sand. Transdermal local anesthetic patches may also provide symptomatic relief in mild cases. If patients do not experience

TABLE 5.1 ■ Differential Diagnosis of Trochanteric Bursitis

- Arthritides of the hip
- Acetabular labral tear
- Avascular necrosis of the femoral head
- Septic arthritis
- Femoroacetabular impingement syndrome
- Fractures of the femoral neck
- Avulsion fractures of the greater trochanter
- Gluteal medius tendinopathy
- Meralgia paresthetica
- Impingement syndromes
- Piriformis tendinopathy
- Piriformis syndrome
- Iliopsoas tendinopathy
- Iliotibial band inflammation
- Snapping hip syndrome
- Legg-Calvé-Perthes disease
- Lumbar radiculopathy
- Complex regional pain syndrome

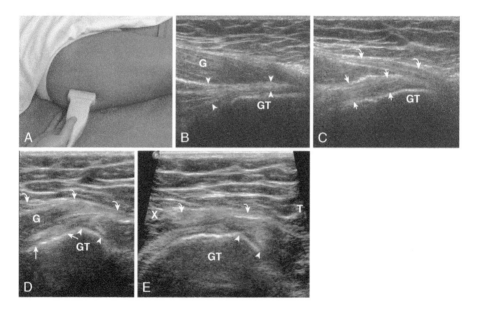

Fig. 5.9 Greater trochanter evaluation. (A) Coronal-oblique imaging over the greater trochanter shows from anterior to posterior (B) the gluteus minimus *(arrowheads)* insertion on the anterior facet of the greater trochanter *(GT)* and (C) the gluteus medius *(arrows)* insertion on the lateral facet of the greater trochanter. Note the iliotibial tract *(curved arrow)* in (C). Transverse images, superior (D) and inferior (E), show, from anterior to posterior, the gluteus minimus attachment *(arrowheads)*, the gluteus medius attachment *(arrows)*, and the iliotibial tract *(curved arrows)*. *G*, Gluteus medius muscle; *T*, tensor fasciae latae; *X*, gluteus maximus. (From Jacobson JA. *Fundamentals of Musculoskeletal Ultrasound.* Philadelphia: Saunders; 2007.)

rapid improvement, injection is a reasonable next step. Ultrasound guidance may improve the accuracy of needle placement in selected patients (Fig. 5.9).

Physical modalities, including local heat and gentle stretching exercises, should be introduced several days after the patient undergoes injection. Vigorous exercises should be avoided because they will exacerbate the patient's symptoms. Simple analgesics, NSAIDs, and antimyotonic agents can be used concurrently with this injection technique.

HIGH-YIELD TAKEAWAYS

- The patient is afebrile, making an acute infectious etiology (e.g., septic arthritis) unlikely.
- The patient's symptomatology is the result of acute trauma and physical examination, and testing should be focused on the identification of ligamentous injury, acute arthritis, tendinitis, and bursitis.
- The patient has point tenderness over the trochanteric bursa, which is highly suggestive of trochanteric bursitis.
- There is warmth and swelling of the area overlying the greater trochanter suggestive of an inflammatory process.
- The patient's symptoms are unilateral and involve only one joint, which is more suggestive of a local process than a systemic polyarthropathy.
- Sleep disturbance is common and must be addressed concurrently with the patient's pain symptomatology.
- Plain radiographs will provide high-yield information regarding the bony contents of the joint and the identification of fractures or other bony abnormalities of the femur as well as calcification of the bursa and tendons, but ultrasound imaging and MRI will be more useful in identifying soft tissue pathology.

Suggested Readings

Waldman SD. Injection Technique for Trochanteric Bursitis. In: *Pain Review*. 2nd ed. Philadelphia: Elsevier; 2017:515–516.

Waldman SD. The Trochanteric Bursa. *Pain Review*. 2nd ed. Philadelphia: Elsevier; 2017:303–304.

Waldman SD. Trochanteric Bursitis and Other Disorders of the Trochanteric Bursa. In: *Waldman's Comprehensive Atlas of Diagnostic Ultrasound of Painful Conditions*. Philadelphia: Wolters Kluwer; 2016:206–215.

Waldman SD. Trochanteric Bursitis Injection. In: *Atlas of Pain Management Injection Techniques*. 4th ed. Philadelphia: Elsevier; 2017:415–419.

Waldman SD. Ultrasound-guided Injection Technique for Trochanteric Bursitis. In: *Comprehensive Atlas of Ultrasound Guided Pain Management Injection Techniques*. Philadelphia: Lippincott; 2014:810–816.

Carol Kane

A 23-Year-Old Female With Buttock and Posterior Hip Pain

- Learn the common causes of posterior hip and buttock pain.
- Develop an understanding of the bursae of the hip and pelvis.
- Develop an understanding of the causes of ischial bursitis.
- Develop an understanding of the differential diagnosis of ischial bursitis.
- Learn the clinical presentation of ischial bursitis.
- Learn how to examine the hip and associated bursae.
- Learn how to use physical examination to identify ischial bursitis.
- Develop an understanding of the treatment options for ischial bursitis.

Carol "Candy" Kane

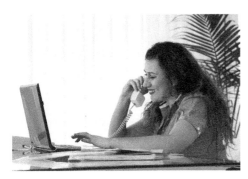

"Hello, Doctor, my name is Carol Kane, but my friends all call me Candy." Carol "Candy" Kane is a 23-year-old receptionist with the chief complaint of, "I've got a pain in my butt." Carol stated that she works as a receptionist for a local interior design firm and was in her usual good state of health until the firm decided to remodel the reception area and replaced her usual chair and desk with a glass-topped table that was "just too high. I was fine with my old chair and desk, but as you can see, I am really short, so the only way I can reach to use my laptop is to sit on the edge of my new chair—and that's been a problem because the edge of the chair is hard, which is what I think is killing my butt. I've tried sitting on a pillow, but the boss doesn't like me doing that because it sends the wrong message to our customers. I asked her if they would buy me a standing desk and they said that didn't match the aesthetic narrative of the firm."

"Carol—or, I'm sorry, Candy, have you ever had anything like this before?" She just shook her head no. She said she had tried taking Motrin and Tylenol, which only provided a little relief. The heating pad made the pain worse, and she volunteered that ice packs only made her cold, but provided no help. She stated that she had a pretty long commute and that driving was getting to be a problem because she had to sit on the right side of her butt to take the weight off the sore spot, making it difficult to use the clutch. By the time she got home, her back and her left buttock was killing her. Candy said that the left part of her butt felt kind of warm and swollen. I asked Candy what made her pain worse and she said, "Anything that involves sitting." As a tear ran down her cheek, Candy said, "Doctor, I really need this job, but my butt really hurts and the pain is messing with my sleep. Every time I roll over, the pain wakes me up. My boyfriend doesn't want to stay over because he says I keep waking him up and he needs his sleep."

I asked Candy to point with one finger to show me where it hurt the most. She stood up, turned around, bent forward, and pointed to a spot just over her left ischial tuberosity and said, "Doctor, this is where it hurts!"

On physical examination, Candy was afebrile. Her respirations were 18 and her pulse was 64 and regular. Her blood pressure was 118/68. Her head, eyes, ears, nose, throat (HEENT) exam was normal, as was her cardiopulmonary

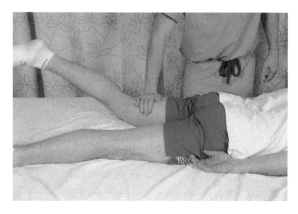

Fig. 6.1   The resisted hip extension test for ischial bursitis. (Courtesy Steven D. Waldman, MD.)

examination. Her thyroid was normal. Her abdominal examination revealed no abnormal mass or organomegaly. There was no costovertebral angle (CVA) tenderness. There was no peripheral edema. Her low back examination was unremarkable. Visual inspection of the area over the left ischial tuberosity revealed mild swelling and felt "boggy" on gentle palpation. The area was warm, but did not appear to be infected. There was marked point tenderness over the left ischial tuberosity. Deep palpation of the area of Candy's pain as well as passive extension of the hip exacerbated the pain. I performed a resisted hip extension test, which was markedly positive on the left and negative on the right (Fig. 6.1). The right hip examination was normal, as was examination of her other major joints. Rectal and pelvic examinations were normal, other than pain with palpation of the left ischial bursa. A careful neurologic examination of the upper and lower extremities revealed there was no evidence of peripheral or entrapment neuropathy, and the deep tendon reflexes were normal.

Key Clinical Points—What's Important and What's Not

THE HISTORY

- Acute onset of left buttock and posterior hip pain attributed to sitting on the edge of a new task chair at work
- Pain localized to the area of the left ischial tuberosity
- Pain exacerbated by sitting
- No other specific traumatic event to the area identified
- No fever or chills
- Sleep disturbance
- Difficulty sitting for any length of time

THE PHYSICAL EXAMINATION

- The patient is afebrile
- Point tenderness to palpation of the area over the ischial tuberosity
- Palpation of the area reveals warmth to touch
- There is swelling and "bogginess" over the left ischial tuberosity
- No evidence of infection
- Pain on extension of the left hip
- The resisted hip extension test was positive on the left (see Fig. 6.1)

OTHER FINDINGS OF NOTE

- Normal HEENT examination
- Normal cardiovascular examination
- Normal pulmonary examination
- Normal abdominal examination
- Normal rectal and pelvic examination
- No peripheral edema
- Normal upper and lower extremity neurologic examination, motor and sensory examination
- Examinations of joints other than the left hip were normal

 What Tests Would You Like to Order?

The following tests were ordered:
- Plain radiographs of the left hip and pelvis
- Ultrasound of the left hip and area over the ischial tuberosity

TEST RESULTS

The plain radiographs of the left hip were reported as normal. Specifically, there was no calcification in the area of the ischial bursa suggestive of chronic bursitis. Ultrasound examination of the left hip was normal, but there was an effusion around the left ischial bursa (Fig. 6.2).

 Clinical Correlation—Putting It All Together

What is the diagnosis?
- Ischial bursitis

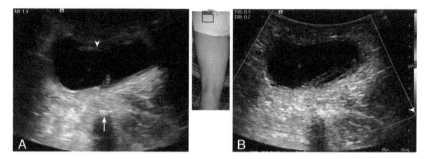

Fig. 6.2   A 75-year-old man reported a painful mass in his right buttock, making it impossible for him to sit down. (A) Ultrasonography shows a cystic lesion *(arrowhead)* over the ischial tuberosity *(arrow)* region. (B) Color Doppler ultrasonography shows minimal vascularity in the wall of the cyst; ischial bursitis was considered. The fluid was aspirated, and a mixture of steroid and lidocaine was injected into the space. This treatment cured the ischial bursitis. (From Chiou H-J, Chou Y-H, Wang H-K, et al. Chronic musculoskeletal pain: ultrasound guided pain control. *Acta Anaesthesiol Taiwan*. 2014;52[3]: 114−133.)

The Science Behind the Diagnosis

ANATOMY

The ischial bursa lies between the gluteus maximus muscle and the ischial tuberosity. It is superior and medial to the insertion of the hamstring muscle onto the ischium (Fig. 6.3). The action of the gluteus maximus muscle includes the flexion of trunk on thigh when maintaining a sitting position, as when riding a horse. This action can irritate the ischial bursa, as can repeated pressure against the bursa that forces it against the ischial tuberosity. The hamstring muscles find a common origin at the ischial tuberosity and can also be irritated from overuse or misuse. The action of the hamstrings includes flexion of the lower extremity at the knee. Running on soft or uneven surfaces can cause a tendinitis at the origin of the hamstring muscles.

CLINICAL SYNDROME

Bursae are formed from synovial sacs, whose purpose is to allow the easy sliding of muscles and tendons across one another at areas of repetitive movement. Lining these synovial sacs is a synovial membrane invested with a network of blood vessels that secrete synovial fluid. With overuse or misuse, the bursa may become inflamed or, rarely, infected; inflammation of the bursa results in an increase in the production of synovial fluid, causing swelling of the bursal sac. Although there is significant interpatient variability in the number, size, and location of bursae, the ischial bursa

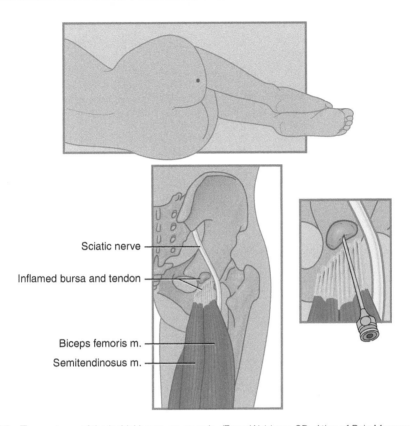

Fig. 6.3 The anatomy of the ischial bursa. *m*, muscle. (From Waldman SD. *Atlas of Pain Management Injection Techniques*. 4th ed. St Louis: Elsevier; 2017: Fig. 112-3.)

generally lies between the gluteus maximus muscle and the bone of the ischial tuberosity. It may exist as a single bursal sac or, in some patients, as a multisegmented series of loculated sacs.

The ischial bursa is vulnerable to injury from both acute trauma and repeated microtrauma. Acute injuries are often caused by direct trauma to the bursa from falls onto the buttock and from overuse, such as prolonged sitting as well as the prolonged riding of horses or bicycles. Running on uneven or soft surfaces such as sand also may cause ischial bursitis (Fig. 6.4). If inflammation of the ischial bursa becomes chronic, calcification may occur.

SIGNS AND SYMPTOMS

Patients suffering from ischial bursitis frequently complain of pain at the base of the buttock with resisted extension of the lower extremity (see Fig. 6.1). The pain is localized to the area over the ischial tuberosity; referred pain is noted in the hamstring muscle, which may develop coexistent tendinitis. Often, patients are

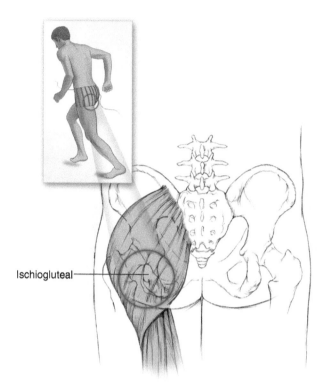

Ischiogluteal

Fig. 6.4 Running on uneven or soft surfaces such as sand may cause ischial bursitis. (From Waldman SD. *Atlas of Common Pain Syndromes*. 4th ed. Philadelphia: Elsevier; 2019: Fig. 91.1.)

unable to sleep on the affected hip and may complain of a sharp "catching" sensation when extending and flexing the hip, especially on first awakening. Physical examination may reveal point tenderness over the ischial tuberosity. Passive straight leg raising and active resisted extension of the affected lower extremity reproduce the pain. Sudden release of resistance during this maneuver causes a marked increase in pain; this increase in pain is considered a positive resisted hip extension test, supporting the diagnosis of ischial bursitis.

TESTING

Plain radiographs are indicated in all patients who present with hip pain to rule out occult bony pathology (Fig. 6.5). If bony pathology is identified, computed tomography (CT) scanning may help further delineate the diagnosis (see Fig. 6.5). Based on the patient's clinical presentation, additional testing may be indicated, including complete blood cell count, sedimentation rate, and antinuclear antibody testing. Magnetic resonance imaging

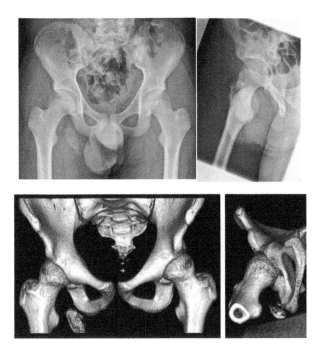

Fig. 6.5 Anteroposterior and lateral radiographs *(upper images)* and computed tomography (3D reconstruction, *lower images*) showing a right ischial tuberosity avulsion fracture. (From Ali AM, Lewis A, Sarraf KM. Surgical treatment of an ischial tuberosity avulsion fracture with delayed presentation. *J Clin Orthop Trauma*. 2020:11[1]:S4—S6 [Fig. 1.1].)

(MRI) or ultrasound imaging of the affected area may also help delineate the presence of other hip bursitis, calcific tendinitis, tendinopathy, triceps tendinitis, or other hip pathology (Figs. 6.6 and 6.7). Rarely, the inflamed bursa may become infected, and failure to diagnose and treat the acute infection can lead to dire consequences.

DIFFERENTIAL DIAGNOSIS

Ischial bursitis is a common cause of hip and groin pain. Table 6.1 lists pathologic conditions that may mimic ischial bursitis. Osteoarthritis, rheumatoid arthritis, posttraumatic arthritis, and (less commonly) aseptic necrosis of the femoral head are also common causes of hip and groin pain that may coexist with ischial bursitis. Hamstring tendinitis or tears of the hamstring muscles may also be present. Less common causes of arthritis-induced pain include the collagen vascular diseases, infection, villonodular synovitis, and Lyme disease. Acute infectious arthritis is usually accompanied by significant systemic symptoms, including fever and malaise, and

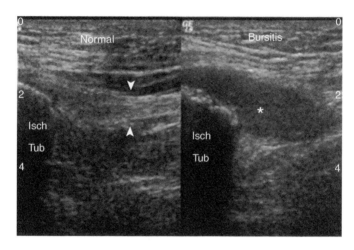

Fig. 6.6 Ischiogluteal bursitis. Longitudinal image at the level of the ischial tuberosity *(Isch Tub)*. Left image demonstrates the normal insertion of the hamstrings tendon *(arrowheads)*. Right image illustrates a distended ischiogluteal bursa *(asterisk)* on the patient's symptomatic side. (From Finlay K, Friedman L. Ultrasonography of the lower extremity. *Orthop Clin North Am.* 2006;37[3]: 245–275.)

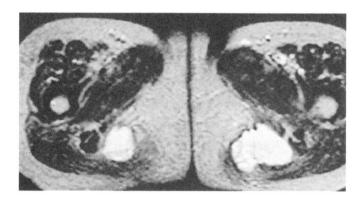

Fig. 6.7 Ischial bursitis: magnetic resonance (MR) imaging. A transaxial T2-weighted (TR/TE, 1500/90) spin-echo MR image shows evidence of bilateral ischial bursitis. (Courtesy J. Dillard MD, San Diego, CA; Resnick D. *Diagnosis of Bone and Joint Disorders.* 4th ed. Philadelphia: Saunders; 2002.)

should be easily recognized; it is treated with culture and antibiotics rather than injection therapy. Collagen vascular disease generally presents as a polyarthropathy rather than a monoarthropathy limited to the hip joint, although pain secondary to collagen vascular disease responds exceedingly well to the injection technique described here.

TABLE 6.1 ■ Differential Diagnosis of Ischial Bursitis

- Hamstring tendinopathy
- Hamstring tears
- Gluteal bursitis
- Avulsion fractures of the ischial tuberosity
- Primary and metastatic tumors involving the ischial tuberosity
- Myofascial pain
- Arthritides of the hip
- Acetabular labral tear
- Avascular necrosis of the femoral head
- Septic arthritis
- Septic bursitis
- Gluteal medius tendinopathy
- Impingement syndromes
- Piriformis tendinopathy
- Piriformis syndrome
- Iliopsoas tendinopathy
- Cluneal nerve entrapment
- Sacroiliac joint dysfunction
- Lumbar spine dysfunction

TREATMENT

Initial treatment of the pain and functional disability associated with ischial bursitis includes a combination of nonsteroidal antiinflammatory drugs (NSAIDs) or cyclooxygenase-2 inhibitors and physical therapy. The local application of heat and cold may also be beneficial. For patients who do not respond to these treatment modalities, injection of local anesthetic and steroid into the ischial bursa is a reasonable next step.

To inject the ischial bursa, the patient is placed in the lateral position with the affected side up and the affected leg flexed at the knee. The skin overlying the ischial tuberosity is prepared with antiseptic solution. A syringe containing 4 mL of 0.25% preservative-free bupivacaine and 40 mg methylprednisolone is attached to a 1.5-inch, 25-gauge needle. The ischial tuberosity is identified with a sterile gloved finger. Before needle placement, the patient should be instructed to say "There!" as soon as a paresthesia is felt in the lower extremity, indicating that the needle has impinged on the sciatic nerve. Should a paresthesia occur, the needle is immediately withdrawn and repositioned more medially. The needle is then carefully advanced through the skin, subcutaneous tissues, muscle, and tendon until it impinges on the bone of the ischial tuberosity (see Fig. 6.3). Care must be taken to keep the needle in the midline and not to advance it laterally, or it could contact the sciatic nerve. After careful aspiration, and if no paresthesia is present, the contents of the syringe are gently injected into the bursa. Ultrasound guidance may improve the accuracy and safety of this technique (Fig. 6.8).

Physical modalities, including local heat and gentle stretching exercises, should be introduced several days after the patient undergoes injection.

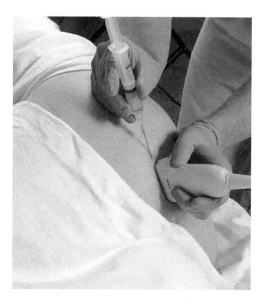

Fig. 6.8 Ultrasound-guided injection of the ischial bursa. (Courtesy Steven D. Waldman MD.)

Vigorous exercises should be avoided, because they will exacerbate the patient's symptoms. Simple analgesics and NSAIDs can be used concurrently with this injection technique.

HIGH-YIELD TAKEAWAYS

- The patient is afebrile, making an acute infectious etiology (e.g., septic arthritis) unlikely.
- The patient's symptomatology is the result of acute trauma and physical examination, and testing should be focused on the identification of ligamentous injury, acute arthritis, tendinitis, and bursitis.
- The patient has point tenderness over the ischial bursa, which is highly suggestive of ischial bursitis.
- There is warmth and swelling of the area overlying the ischial tuberosity, suggestive of an inflammatory process.
- The patient's symptoms are unilateral and involve only one joint, which is more suggestive of a local process than a systemic polyarthropathy.
- Sleep disturbance is common and must be addressed concurrently with the patient's pain symptomatology.

(Continued)

- Plain radiographs will provide high-yield information regarding the bony contents of the joint and the identification of fractures or other bony abnormalities of the femur as well as calcification of the bursa and tendons, but ultrasound imaging and MRI will be more useful in identifying soft tissue pathology.

Suggested Readings

Lormeau C, Cormier G, Sigaux J, et al. Management of septic bursitis. *Joint Bone Spine.* 2018;341−347.

Waldman SD. Injection Technique for Ischial Bursitis. In: *Atlas of Pain Management Injection Techniques.* 4th ed. Philadelphia: Elsevier; 2017:400−404.

Waldman SD. Ischial Bursitis. In: *Atlas of Common Pain Syndromes.* 4th ed. Philadelphia: Elsevier; 2019:395−398.

Waldman SD. Ischial Bursitis. In: *Imaging of Pain.* Philadelphia: Saunders Elsevier; 2011: 349−350.

Waldman SD. Ischial Bursitis. In: *Pain Review.* 2nd ed. Philadelphia: Elsevier; 2017: 510−511.

Waldman SD. Ischial Bursitis. In: *Waldman's Comprehensive Atlas of Diagnostic Ultrasound of Painful Conditions.* Philadelphia: Wolters Kluwer; 2016:455−459.

Wisniewski SJ, Hurdle M, Erickson JM, et al. Ultrasound-guided ischial bursa injection: technique and positioning considerations. *PM&R.* 2014;6(1):56−60.

Jimmie Kaline

A 27-Year-Old Male With a Snapping Hip

LEARNING OBJECTIVES

- Learn the common causes of snapping hip.
- Develop an understanding of the unique anatomy of the hip joint.
- Develop an understanding of the bursae of the hip.
- Develop an understanding of the tendons of the hip.
- Develop an understanding of the causes of snapping hip.
- Develop an understanding of the differential diagnosis of snapping hip.
- Learn the clinical presentation of snapping hip.
- Learn how to examine the hip and associated bursae.
- Learn how to use physical examination to identify snapping hip.
- Develop an understanding of the treatment options for snapping hip.

Jimmie Kaline

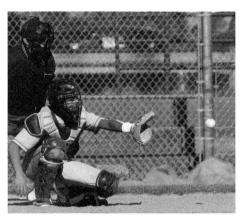

Jimmie Kaline is a 27-year-old minor league baseball player with the chief complaint of, "My left hip keeps snapping." Jimmie stated that ever since spring training, every time that he gets up from behind home plate, his hip snaps. He said that the snap is so loud that the home plate umpire, batter, and the guys in the dugout can hear it, and some of his teammates have taken to call him "Snap, Crackle, and Pop." Jimmie states, "Doctor, this snapping is really driving me crazy! At first it was just the snap, but now my hip has started to hurt. I had really hoped to make it up to the majors this season, but I'm afraid that the snapping sound will make them think I am injured."

I asked Jimmie about any previous injuries to the left hip and he said he couldn't count the number of times he had been hit with thrown bats and wild pitches, but it was just part of the job. He didn't know a baseball catcher who didn't have all kinds of aches and pains. It just went with the territory. During the season, he pretty much lived on Advil and Icy Hot. "Doc, I can tough it through the pain, but the snapping is really freaking me out. What the hell is wrong with my hip?"

I asked Jimmie what made his hip snap, and he said, "Any time I go from squatting to standing, bam! There it is—snap—and then the pain. My left hip aches all the time now; it really hurts and the pain is really messing with my sleep. Every time I roll over onto my left side, the pain in my left hip wakes me up."

I asked Jimmie to point with one finger to show me where the snap came from, and he pointed to the area just over the left greater trochanter. To further illustrate, he dropped into a squat and the jumped back up. Sure enough, as he stood, there was a loud snap!

On physical examination, Jimmie was afebrile. His respirations were 18 and his pulse was 64 and regular. His blood pressure was 118/70. Jimmie's head, eyes, ears, nose, throat (HEENT) exam was normal, as was his cardiopulmonary examination. His thyroid was normal, as was his abdominal examination. There was no costovertebral angle (CVA) tenderness. There was no peripheral edema. His low back examination was unremarkable. Visual inspection of the left lateral hip was unremarkable. The area over the left greater trochanter was warm but did not appear to be infected. There was subtle point tenderness over the greater trochanter, suggestive of a mild trochanteric bursitis. I performed a snap test,

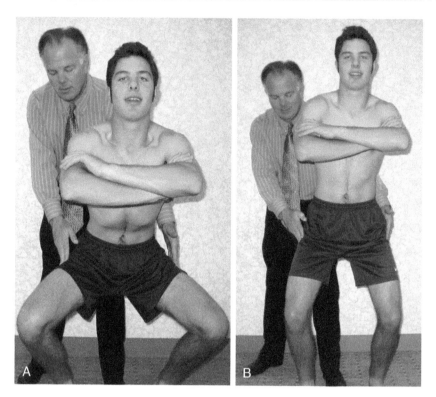

Fig. 7.1 The snap test for snapping hip syndrome is performed by having the patient move rapidly from a squatting (A) to a standing (B) position while the clinician palpates the area over the greater trochanter. (From Waldman SD. *Physical Diagnosis of Pain: An Atlas of Signs and Symptoms*. 3rd ed. St Louis: Elsevier; 2016: Fig. 194-1A,B.)

which was markedly positive on the left and negative on the right (Fig. 7.1). There was both an audible and a palpable snap.

Range of motion of the hip joint, especially resisted abduction of the joint, reproduced Jimmie's pain. The right hip examination was normal, as was examination of his other major joints. A careful neurologic examination of the upper and lower extremities revealed there was no evidence of peripheral or entrapment neuropathy, and the deep tendon reflexes were normal. Specifically, there was no evidence of meralgia paresthetica, which is so common in baseball catchers.

Key Clinical Points—What's Important and What's Not

THE HISTORY

- Onset of an audible snap sound from the left hip pain when rising from a squatting to a standing position

- Pain localized to the area of the left greater trochanter
- Pain associated with a snapping sensation
- No other specific traumatic event to the area identified
- No fever or chills
- Sleep disturbance

THE PHYSICAL EXAMINATION

- The patient is afebrile
- There is an audible and palpable snap when rising from a squatting to a standing position
- Point tenderness to palpation of the area over the trochanteric bursa
- Palpation of the area overlying the left greater trochanter is warm to touch
- No evidence of infection
- Pain on resisted abduction of the affected left hip
- The snap test was positive on the left (see Fig. 7.1)

OTHER FINDINGS OF NOTE

- Normal HEENT examination
- Normal cardiovascular examination
- Normal pulmonary examination
- Normal abdominal examination
- No peripheral edema
- Normal upper and lower extremity neurologic examination, motor and sensory examination
- No evidence of meralgia paresthetica
- Examinations of other joints other than the left hip were normal

 What Tests Would You Like to Order?

The following tests were ordered:
- Plain radiographs of the left hip
- Ultrasound of the left hip and iliotibial band

TEST RESULTS

The plain radiographs of the left hip were reported as normal. Ultrasound examination of the left hip revealed an effusion around the trochanteric bursa and mild displacement of the iliotibial band (Fig. 7.2).

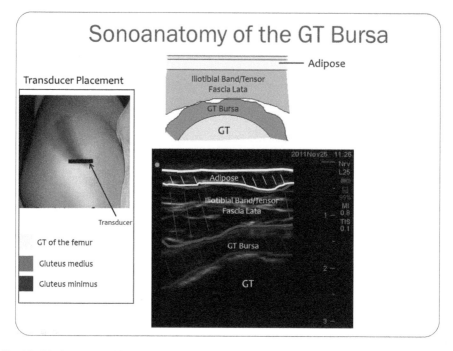

Fig. 7.2   Displacement of iliotibial band. (Courtesy Steven D. Waldman, MD.)

📋 Clinical Correlation—Putting It All Together

What is the diagnosis?
- Snapping hip syndrome

The Science Behind the Diagnosis

ANATOMY

The trochanteric bursa lies between the greater trochanter and the tendon of the gluteus medius and the iliotibial tract (Figs. 7.3 and 7.4). The gluteus medius muscle has its origin from the outer surface of the ilium, and its fibers pass downward and laterally to attach on the lateral surface of the greater trochanter. The gluteus medius locks the pelvis in place when walking and running. The gluteus medius muscle is innervated by the superior gluteal nerve. The iliotibial band is an extension of the fascia lata, which inserts at the lateral condyle of the tibia (Fig. 7.5). The iliotibial band can rub backward and forward over the lateral epicondyle of the femur and irritate the iliotibial bursa beneath it.

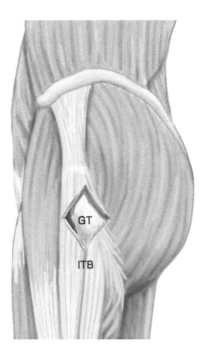

Fig. 7.3 Lateral snapping of the hip can be caused by the iliotibial band (ITB) passing forcefully across the greater trochanter (GT) during forceful hip flexion. (From Waldman SD. *Atlas of Pain Management Injection Techniques*. 4th ed. St Louis: Elsevier; 2017: Fig. 118-2.)

CLINICAL SYNDROME

Snapping hip, which is also known as coxa saltans, is an uncommon cause of lateral hip pain. It is not a single syndrome, but a group of disorders that have in common abnormal passage of musculotendininous units or fascial bands over the greater trochanter. In an effort to better understand the pathophysiology responsible for snapping hip syndrome in a specific patient, it is helpful to classify the pathology as to the anatomic structures or region responsible for the symptomatology (Table 7.1). To this end, snapping hip syndrome can be classified as external, internal, or intraarticular. The pathophysiology associated with external slipping hip syndrome is related to abnormal passage of the posterior border of the iliotibial band or the anterior border of the gluteus maximus muscle over the greater trochanter (see Fig. 7.5). The pathophysiology of internal snapping hip syndrome is thought to be related to the abnormal passage of the psoas tendon over the iliopectineal eminence (Fig. 7.6). Loose bodies, synovial abnormalities, and tears of the labrum have been implicated as the cause of intraarticular snapping hip syndrome (Fig. 7.7).

The constellation of symptoms associated with external snapping hip syndrome includes a snapping, clicking, or grating sensation in the lateral hip

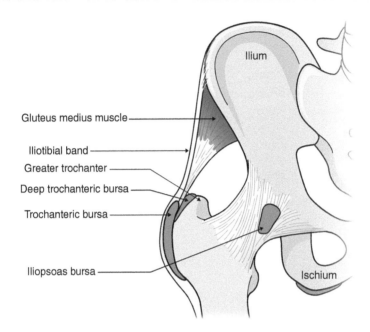

Fig. 7.4 The trochanteric bursa lies between the greater trochanter and the tendon of the gluteus medius and the iliotibial tract. This bursa may exist as a single bursal sac or, in some patients, as a multisegmented series of loculated sacs.

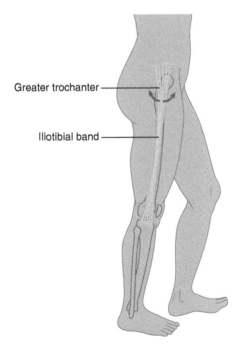

Fig. 7.5 The relationship of the iliotibial band and the greater trochanter. (From Waldman SD. *Atlas of Pain Management Injection Techniques*. 4th ed. St Louis: Elsevier; 2017: Fig. 118-1.)

TABLE 7.1 ■ **Causes of Snapping Hip Syndrome**

External Causes
- Abnormal passage of the iliotibial band over the greater trochanter
- Abnormal passage of the tensor fascia lata over the greater trochanter
- Abnormal passage of the gluteus medius tendon over the greater trochanter
- Snapping hip

Internal Causes
- Abnormal passage of the iliopsoas tendon over the anterior inferior iliac spine
- Abnormal passage of the iliopsoas tendon over the lesser trochanter
- Abnormal passage of the iliopsoas tendon over the iliopectineal ridge

Intraarticular Causes
- Torn acetabular labrum
- Repeated subluxation of the hip
- Torn ligamentum teres
- Synovial chondromatosis
- Joint mice
- Abnormalities of the articular cartilage

associated with sudden, sharp pain in the area of the greater trochanter. The symptomatology of snapping hip syndrome occurs most commonly when the patient rises from a sitting to a standing position or when walking briskly. Often, trochanteric bursitis coexists with snapping hip syndrome, further increasing the patient's pain and disability.

SIGNS AND SYMPTOMS

Patients suffering from external snapping hip syndrome can usually recreate the snapping and pain by moving from a squatting to a standing position and by forcibly adducting the hip. These patients will also usually exhibit a positive snap test. The snap test is performed by having the patient move rapidly from a squatting to a standing position while the clinician palpates the area over the grater trochanter (see Fig. 7.1). Point tenderness over the trochanteric bursa indicative of trochanteric bursitis also is often present.

TESTING

Plain radiographs of the hip may reveal calcification of the bursa and associated structures consistent with chronic inflammation (Fig. 7.8). Magnetic resonance imaging (MRI) and ultrasound imaging are indicated if occult mass or tumor of the hip or groin is suspected or to confirm the diagnosis (Fig. 7.9). Dynamic ultrasound imaging of the region of the greater trochanter while flexing and extending the hip may demonstrate the snapping of

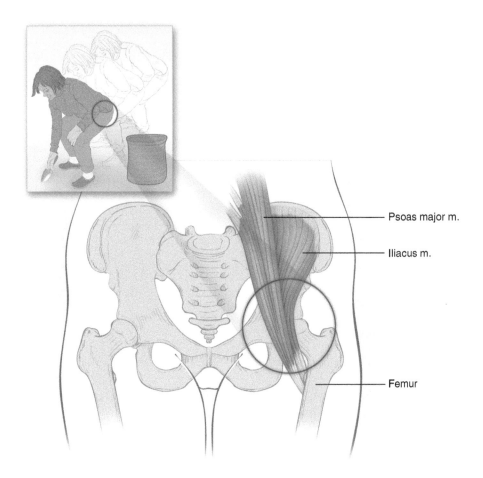

Fig. 7.6 The pathophysiology of internal snapping hip syndrome is thought to be related to the abnormal passage of the psoas tendon over the iliopectineal eminence. *m*, muscle. (From Waldman SD. *Atlas of Common Pain Syndromes*. 4th ed. Philadelphia: Elsevier; 2019: Fig. 99.2.)

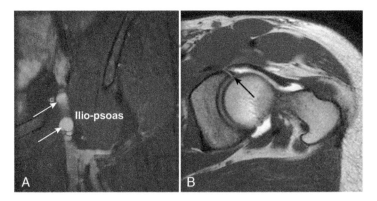

Fig. 7.7 (A, B) Loose bodies, synovial abnormalities, and tears of the labrum have been implicated as the cause of intraarticular snapping hip syndrome. (From Waldman SD, Campbell RSD. *Imaging of Pain*. Philadelphia: Saunders; 2011: Fig. 136.2.)

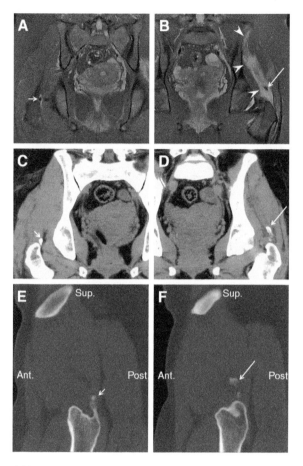

Fig 7.8 A 33-year-old female with a 1-day history of low back, buttock, and posterolateral thigh pain on left (B, D, and F); images illustrate concurrent asymptomatic calcific deposit in the superoposterior tendon of the right gluteus medius (A, C, and E). Fat-suppressed proton density coronal magnetic resonance (MR) images with effusion *(arrowheads)* surrounding the left gluteus medius muscle and low signal calcifications *(arrow)* in the tendon (B). On asymptomatic right side (A), note intratendinous calcification as low signal area with high signal rim *(small arrow)* but no muscle edema or effusion. Coronal and sagittal computed tomography (CT) images depicting well-circumscribed asymptomatic calcification *(small arrows)* of homogeneous density (C, E) and symptomatic calcifications *(arrows)* with fluffy, ill-defined edges (D, F) in the superoposterior tendons of the gluteus medius, bilaterally. (From Paik NC. Acute calcific tendinitis of the gluteus medius: an uncommon source for back, buttock, and thigh pain. *Sem Arthr Rheum.* 2014;43[6]:824–829 [Fig. 2].)

the iliotibial band over the greater trochanter (Fig. 7.10). A complete blood count and erythrocyte sedimentation rate are useful if infection is suspected. Electromyography can distinguish snapping hip from meralgia paresthetica and sciatica. Injection of the area of the trochanteric bursa with local anesthetic and steroid may serve as both a diagnostic and a therapeutic maneuver.

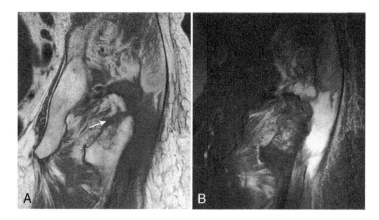

Fig. 7.9 (A) Coronal T1-weighted (T1W) magnetic resonance (MR) image of an elderly woman with osteoporosis and lateral hip pain but no history of trauma. Previous radiographic findings had been normal. There is an insufficiency fracture through the base of the greater trochanter *(white arrow)*. (B) The coronal fat-suppressed T2-weighted (FST2W) MR image shows the extensive high signal intensity hematoma within the adjacent trochanteric bursa, with more generalized soft tissue edema. The fracture line is not well shown, but there is marrow edema in the proximal femur. (From Waldman SD, Campbell RSD. *Imaging of Pain*. Philadelphia: Saunders; 2011: Fig. 142.5.)

DIFFERENTIAL DIAGNOSIS

The diagnosis of snapping hip syndrome is based on clinical findings rather than specific laboratory, electrodiagnostic, or radiographic testing. For this reason, a targeted history and physical examination, with a systematic search for other causes of hip pain, should be carried out. It is incumbent on the clinician to rule out other coexisting disease processes that may mimic snapping hip syndrome, including primary inflammatory muscle disease, primary hip pathology, and rectal and pelvic tumors. Snapping hip syndrome frequently coexists with trochanteric bursitis and arthritis of the hip, which may require specific treatment to provide palliation of pain and return of function. Occasionally, snapping hip syndrome can be confused with meralgia paresthetica because both manifest with pain in the lateral thigh. The two syndromes can be distinguished by the fact that patients with meralgia paresthetica do not have any of the previously mentioned physical findings associated with snapping hip syndrome and have decreased sensation in the distribution of the lateral femoral cutaneous nerve. Causes of snapping hip are listed in Table 7.1.

TREATMENT

A short course of conservative therapy consisting of simple analgesics, nonsteroidal antiinflammatory drugs (NSAIDs), or cyclooxygenase-2 inhibitors is a reasonable first step in the treatment of snapping hip. Patients should be

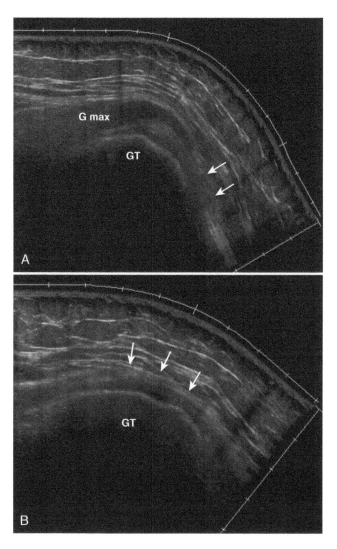

Fig. 7.10 Transverse ultrasound (US) images of a patient with symptoms of a snapping hip. Magnetic resonance imaging (MRI) findings were unremarkable. (A) In flexion, the anterior leading edge of the gluteus maximus *(G max)* extends around the lateral margin of the greater trochanter *(GT)*, with the echo-bright iliotibial band (ITB) anteriorly *(white arrows)*. (B) In extension, the gluteus maximus moves posteriorly and the ITB *(white arrows)* lies against the lateral margin of the GT. Dynamic US showed that this action did not occur smoothly, but the ITB snapped back suddenly into position as the leg neared full extension. (From Waldman SD, Campbell RSD. *Imaging of Pain*. Philadelphia: Saunders; 2011: Fig. 143.2.)

instructed to avoid repetitive activities that may be responsible for the development of snapping hip, such as running on sand. Transdermal local anesthetic patches may also provide symptomatic relief in mild cases. If patients do not experience rapid improvement, injection is a reasonable next step.

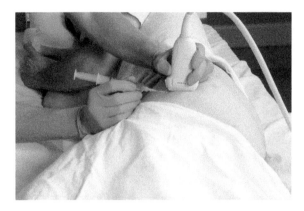

Fig. 7.11 Correct in-plane needle placement for ultrasound-guided injection of the area of the trochanteric bursa. (Courtesy Steven D. Waldman, MD.)

Ultrasound guidance may improve the accuracy of needle placement in selected patients (Fig. 7.11).

Physical modalities, including local heat and gentle stretching exercises, should be introduced several days after the patient undergoes injection. Vigorous exercises should be avoided, because they will exacerbate the patient's symptoms. Simple analgesics, NSAIDs, and antimyotonic agents can be used concurrently with this injection technique.

HIGH-YIELD TAKEAWAYS

- The patient is afebrile, making an acute infectious etiology (e.g., septic arthritis, bursitis, or osteomyelitis) unlikely.
- The patient's symptomatology is the likely result of chronic overuse and irritation of the iliotibial band and tensor fascia lata.
- Since snapping hip is a clinical diagnosis, physical examination and testing should be focused not only on the identification of ligamentous injury, acute arthritis, tendinitis, and bursitis, but also on other pathologic processes that have the potential to harm the patient (osteomyelitis, osseous tumors, sarcomas, etc.).
- The patient has an audible and palpable snap when rising from a squatting to a standing position, which is highly suggestive of snapping hip.
- There is warmth and swelling of the area overlying the greater trochanter, suggestive of an inflammatory process.

(Continued)

- The patient has point tenderness over the trochanteric bursa, which is highly suggestive of trochanteric bursitis, which frequently coexists with snapping hip syndrome.
- The patient's symptoms are unilateral and involve only one joint, which is more suggestive of a local process than a systemic polyarthropathy.
- Plain radiographs will provide high-yield information regarding the bony contents of the joint and the identification of fractures or other bony abnormalities of the femur as well as calcification of the bursa and tendons, but ultrasound imaging and MRI will be more useful in identifying soft tissue pathology.
- Dynamic ultrasound imaging may provide identification of the specific anatomic structures responsible for the snap.

Suggested Readings

Waldman SD. Snapping Hip and Other Disorders of the Trochanteric Bursa. In: *Waldman's Comprehensive Atlas of Diagnostic Ultrasound of Painful Conditions*. Philadelphia: Wolters Kluwer; 2016:717−724.

Waldman SD. Snapping Hip Injection. In: *Atlas of Pain Management Injection Techniques*. 4th ed. Philadelphia: Elsevier; 2017:424−429.

Waldman SD. The Trochanteric Bursa. In: *Pain Review*. 2nd ed. Philadelphia: Elsevier; 2017:303−304.

Waldman SD. Ultrasound-guided Injection Technique for Snapping Hip. In: *Waldman's Comprehensive Atlas of Ultrasound Guided Pain Management Injection Techniques*. Philadelphia: Lippincott; 2014:817−821.

Waldman SD, Campbell RSD. Snapping Hip Syndrome. In: *Imaging of Pain*. Philadelphia: Saunders; 2011:365−366.

Zoey Hart

A 25-Year-Old Female With Suprapubic Pain

LEARNING OBJECTIVES

- Learn the common causes of groin pain.
- Develop an understanding of the anatomy of the nerves of the groin and pelvis.
- Develop an understanding of the anatomy of the symphysis pubis.
- Develop an understanding of the causes of osteitis pubis.
- Learn the clinical presentation of osteitis pubis.
- Learn how to use physical examination to identify osteitis pubis.
- Develop an understanding of the treatment options for osteitis pubis.
- Learn the appropriate testing options to help diagnose osteitis pubis.
- Learn to identify red flags in patients who present with groin pain.
- Develop an understanding of the role in interventional pain management in the treatment of osteitis pubis.

Zoey Hart

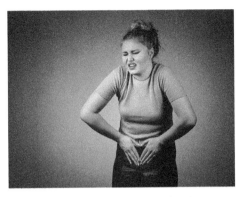

Zoey Hart is a 25-years-old physical therapist with the chief complaint of, "I've got pain in my suprapubic region ever since my C-section." Zoey went on to say that she had a bad urinary tract infection following the placement of a urinary catheter that was a real pistol to get rid of. "I took six different antibiotics before we got a handle on it. It made the first few weeks at home a real nightmare. No breast feeding, constantly getting up to pee—it was no fun at all." I asked if Zoey knew what they cultured and she said that her cultures never grew anything, which made it all the more frustrating. "The UTI symptoms are better, but I am still having a lot of suprapubic pain. I feel like the pain is making me walk funny. My gait is really off, so I have to waddle like a duck."

I asked Zoey if she had any fever or chills with her urinary tract infection and she shook her head and said that she didn't think so. "I just had to pee about 500 times a day." I asked Zoey if this was her first child and she smiled brightly and said, "Yes, and she is a real angel! Doctor, it's been great except for this pain. At first I thought it was just a combination of the UTI and post-C-section pain, but as I healed up, the suprapubic pain just didn't go away. The pain and the crazy walking thing have made it really hard to get back in shape and lose weight."

I asked Zoey if she had ever had anything like this before and she shook her head no. She also denied any current urinary or gynecologic symptoms, hematuria, or fever or chills. She also denied a history of kidney stones. She had started her periods again with her last menstrual period a week ago. Zoey was using oral contraceptives, but volunteered that the pelvic pain made sex pretty unpleasant. I asked what she was doing to manage the pain and she said that "nothing really works." I asked her to rate her pain on a scale of 1 to 10, with 10 being the worst pain she had ever had. She said the pain was a 7 or 8. "Doctor, if I have to live with the pain, I can, but it is interfering with everything—getting dressed, walking, exercise, taking care of my daughter, sex—everything. I just really need to get my life back on track."

I asked Zoey to point with one finger to show me where it hurt the most. She pointed to her suprapubic area and said, "Doc, the pain is right here. The C-section incision is all healed up and although I won't be wearing a bikini any time soon, it really doesn't hurt, but there is this spot right here in the center right over my pubic bone that is really killing me."

On physical examination, Zoey was afebrile. Her respirations were 16. Her pulse was 72 and regular. Her blood pressure (BP) was normal at 112/72. Her head, eyes, ears, nose, throat (HEENT) exam was normal, as was her thyroid examination. Her cardiopulmonary examination was negative. Her abdominal examination revealed no abnormal mass or organomegaly. There was no costo-vertebral angle (CVA) tenderness. There was no peripheral edema. Her low back examination was unremarkable. Her lower extremity neurologic examina-tion was completely normal. I asked Zoey to lie back on the examination table with her knees bent so we could take a closer look at her cesarean section scar. Visual inspection of the scar revealed no obvious defect or infection. Inspection of the groin revealed no obvious abnormal mass or inguinal hernia. I again asked Zoey to use one finger to point to the spot that hurt, and she care-fully pointed to a spot overlying the pubic symphysis (Fig. 8.1). I asked Zoey if I could palpate the spot she identified, and after a moment's hesitation she nod-ded yes and said, "Sure, but be gentle. It really is sensitive." I said, "No problem, why don't you hold my hand and you do the pushing and I'll do the feeling and together we'll figure out what is going on." She liked that idea and I had Zoey guide my index finger to the spot that was causing the trouble. The spot was right over the symphysis pubis, and when Zoey tentatively pushed my index fin-ger a little harder, I felt her suddenly withdraw her pelvis as she said, "Right there!" I said, "I think I know what's going on. How about getting up and walking down the hall for me?" She carefully sat up and slid off the exam table. As she took off down the hall, I immediately noticed a waddling gait and I was pretty sure that I had my answer as to what was causing Zoey's pain and physi-cal disability (Fig. 8.2).

Key Clinical Points—What's Important and What's Not
THE HISTORY

- A history of the recent onset of suprapubic pain following a cesarean section, which was complicated by persistent urinary tract infections
- No history of gynecologic symptoms related to the pain
- No history of kidney stones
- No history of hematuria
- Difficulty in ambulating without suprapubic pain
- Abnormal waddling gait noted by patient
- Pain is localized to symphysis pubis
- No fever or chills

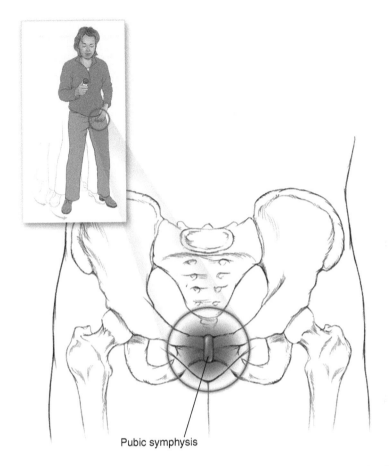

Pubic symphysis

Fig. 8.1 The pain of osteitis pubis is localized to the symphysis pubis with occasional radiation into the inner thighs. (From Waldman SD. *Atlas of Common Pain Syndromes*. 4th ed. Philadelphia: Elsevier; 2019: Fig. 88.2.)

THE PHYSICAL EXAMINATION

- The patient is afebrile
- Normal visual inspection of the cesarean section scar
- Palpation of the symphysis pubis elicits pain
- Patient has waddling gait (see Fig. 8.2)
- The lower extremity neurologic examination is within normal limits

OTHER FINDINGS OF NOTE

- Normal BP
- Normal HEENT examination
- Normal cardiopulmonary examination

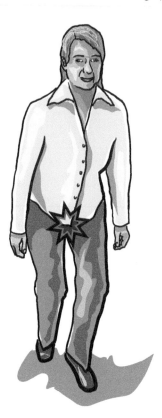

Fig. 8.2 Patients suffering from osteitis pubis will often develop a waddling gait in an effort to splint the symphysis pubis. (From Waldman SD. *Physical Diagnosis of Pain: An Atlas of Signs and Symptoms*. 3rd ed. St Louis: Elsevier; 2016: Fig. 162-3.)

- Normal abdominal examination
- No peripheral edema
- No groin mass or inguinal hernia
- No CVA tenderness

 ## What Tests Would You Like to Order?

The following tests were ordered:
- X-ray of pelvis with special attention to the symphysis pubis
- Magnetic resonance imaging (MRI) of the pelvis with special attention to the symphysis pubis

TEST RESULTS

Plain radiograph of the pelvis demonstrates noninfectious changes of the symphysis pubis consistent with osteitis pubis (Fig. 8.3). MRI of the pelvis reveals high signal intensity marrow edema in both pubic bones as well as periosteal edema consistent with osteitis pubis (Fig. 8.4).

Clinical Correlation—Putting It All Together

What is the diagnosis?
- Osteitis pubis

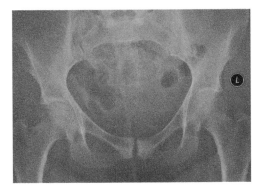

Fig. 8.3 Plain radiograph of the pelvis demonstrates noninfectious changes of the symphysis pubis, consistent with osteitis pubis. *L*, Left. (From Waldman SD, Campbell RSD. *Imaging of Pain*. Philadelphia: Saunders; 2011; Fig. 82-1.)

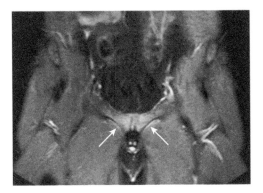

Fig. 8.4 Coronal stir magnetic resonance (MR) image demonstrates high signal intensity marrow edema in both pubic bones *(arrows)* as well as periosteal edema consistent with osteitis pubis. (From Waldman SD, Campbell RSD. *Imaging of Pain*. Philadelphia: Saunders; 2011: Fig. 82-2.)

The Science Behind the Diagnosis

ANATOMY OF THE SYMPHYSIS PUBIS

The symphysis pubis is a nonsynovial amphiarthrodial joint that provides articulation between the two pubic bones. The avascular interpubic fibroelastic cartilage connects the two opposing articular surfaces of the pubic bones (Fig. 8.5). The interpubic fibroelastic cartilage is wider anteriorly, narrowing toward the back of the joint space. This asymmetric shape gives the joint space and its adjacent pubic bodies their characteristic heart-shaped appearance on transverse ultrasound scan (see Fig. 8.7). These articular surfaces have thin layers of hyaline articular cartilage that are subject to damage or inflammation. In health, the joint can be moved forward and backward approximately 2 mm with a minimal amount of rotation. The range of motion of the joint increases dramatically in women during childbirth. The joint is relatively avascular, which accounts for the difficulty in treating joint space infections of the symphysis pubis. The joint is strengthened by a variety of ligaments, including the superior pubic ligament, which connects the top of the joint, and the arcuate ligament, which strengthens the joint from below. These ligaments as well as the anterior

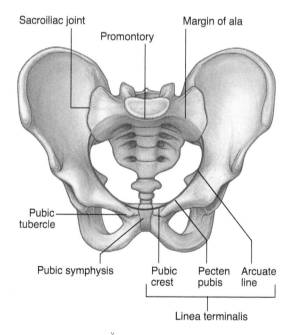

Fig. 8.5 The symphysis pubis. (From Vodušek D, Boller F. Neurology of sexual and bladder disorders. In: *Handbook of Clinical Neurology*. Amsterdam: Elsevier; 2015: Fig. 2.)

and posterior aponeuroses are subject to disruption from blunt trauma to the pelvis, including seatbelt injuries (Fig. 8.6).

CLINICAL SYNDROME

Osteitis pubis causes localized tenderness over the symphysis pubis, pain radiating into the inner thigh, and a waddling gait. Radiographic changes consisting of erosion, sclerosis, and widening of the symphysis pubis are pathognomonic for osteitis pubis (see Fig. 8.3). This is a disease of the second through fourth decades, and girls and women are affected more frequently than are boys and men. Osteitis pubis occurs most commonly after bladder, inguinal, or prostate surgery, and is thought to result from the hematogenous spread of infection to the relatively avascular symphysis pubis. Osteitis pubis can also occur without an obvious inciting factor or infection (Box 8.1).

SIGNS AND SYMPTOMS

On physical examination, patients exhibit point tenderness over the symphysis pubis, and the pain may radiate into the inner thigh with palpation of the symphysis pubis. Patients may also have tenderness over the anterior pelvis. The pain of osteitis pubis is aggravated by running, kicking, pivoting on one leg, and lying on the side. Patients often adopt a waddling gait to avoid movement of the symphysis pubis (see Fig. 8.2). This dysfunctional gait may result in lower extremity bursitis and tendinitis, which can confuse the clinical picture and add to the patient's pain and disability.

TESTING

Plain radiography is indicated in all patients who present with pain thought to be emanating from the symphysis pubis to rule out occult bony disorders and tumor (Fig. 8.7). Based on the patient's clinical presentation, additional testing may be warranted, including a complete blood count, prostate-specific antigen level, erythrocyte sedimentation rate, C-reactive protein, serum protein electrophoresis, and antinuclear antibody testing. Magnetic resonance imaging (MRI) and ultrasound imaging of the pelvis are indicated if occult mass or tumor is suspected (Figs. 8.8 and 8.9). Radionuclide bone scanning may be useful to identify inflammation and to exclude stress fractures not visible on plain radiographs (Fig. 8.10). The injection technique described later serves as both a diagnostic and a therapeutic maneuver.

A

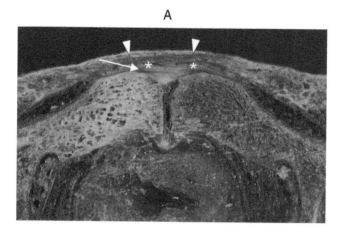

B

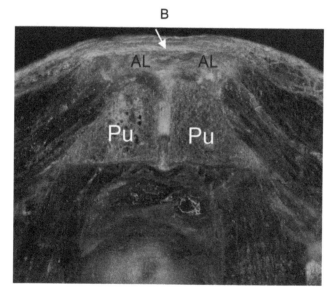

Fig. 8.6 The symphysis pubis. (A) At level 2, the anterior *(arrowheads)* and posterior aponeurosis *(arrow)* are seen. Note pyramidalis muscles in between *(asterisk)*. (B) At level 3, the bulk of the adductor longus tendons is seen *(AL)* inserting on the pubic bone and cross-connecting via the anterior pubic ligament *(arrow)*. *Pu,* pubic bone. (From De Maeseneer M, Forsyth R, Provyn S, et al. MR imaging-anatomical-histological evaluation of the abdominal muscles, aponeurosis, and adductor tendon insertions on the pubic symphysis: a cadaver study. *Eur J Radiol.* 2019;118:107−113 [Fig. 3].)

DIFFERENTIAL DIAGNOSIS

A pain syndrome that is clinically similar to osteitis pubis may occur in patients with rheumatoid arthritis or ankylosing spondylitis; however, the characteristic radiographic changes of osteitis pubis are lacking. Adductor muscle strain and

BOX 8.1 ■ Causes of Osteitis Pubis

- Suprapubic gynecologic surgeries
- Suprapubic urologic surgeries
- Groin surgeries
- Athletic injuries (especially Australian football)
- Pregnancy/childbirth
- Blunt trauma to the pubic symphysis, including seatbelt injuries
- Repetitive stress injuries from running on uneven surfaces
- Leg length discrepancies

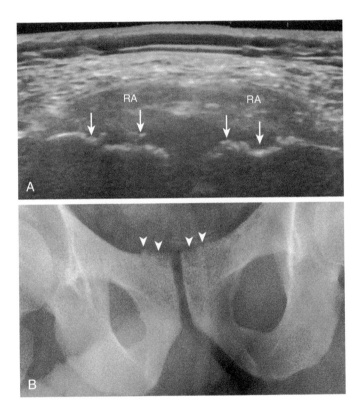

Fig. 8.7 A 34-year-old male recreational athlete with groin pain (diagnosed as osteitis pubis). (A) Panoramic ultrasound imaging with sonopalpation clearly showing the cortical lesions in detail *(arrows)*. (B) Small irregularities *(arrowheads)* on the anteroposterior X-ray film were also suggestive of the diagnosis. *RA,* Rectus abdominis muscle. (From Özçakar L, Utku B. Ultrasound images of groin pain in the athlete: a pictorial essay. *PMR.* 2014;6:753–756.)

avulsion fractures may mimic the presentation of osteitis pubis. Multiple myeloma and metastatic tumor may also mimic the pain and radiographic changes of osteitis pubis. Insufficiency fractures of the pubic rami should be considered if generalized osteoporosis is present.

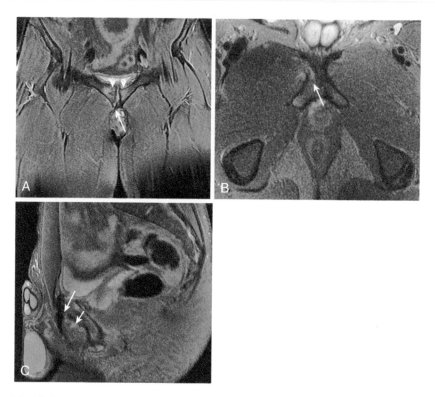

Fig. 8.8 (A) Coronal fat saturated T2-weighted magnetic resonance (MR) image. Bilateral osteitis pubis, right worse than left, characterized by bone marrow hyperintensity *(arrowheads)*, with microtearing along the medial right obturator externus attachment and disruption of the prepubic aponeurotic complex causing secondary cleft formation *(arrow)*. (B) Axial fat saturated T2-weighted MR image demonstrating microtearing of the right obturator externus attachment posterior to the adductor longus with secondary bony stress reaction *(arrow)*. (C) Sagittal fat-saturated T2-weighted MR image. Edema and microtearing of the origin of the obturator externus *(short arrow)* posterior to adductor longus and brevis, extending posterior to the adductor longus origin from the prepubic aponeurotic complex *(long arrow)*. (From MacMahon PJ, Hogan BA, Shelly MJ, et al. Imaging of groin pain. *Magn Reson Imaging Clin N Am.* 2009;17:655–666.)

TREATMENT

Initial treatment of the pain and functional disability associated with osteitis pubis includes a combination of nonsteroidal antiinflammatory drugs (NSAIDs) or cyclooxygenase-2 inhibitors and physical therapy. The local application of heat and cold may also be beneficial. For patients who do not respond to these treatment modalities, injection with local anesthetic and steroid is a reasonable next step.

Injection for osteitis pubis is carried out by placing the patient in the supine position. The midpoints of the pubic bones and the symphysis pubis are

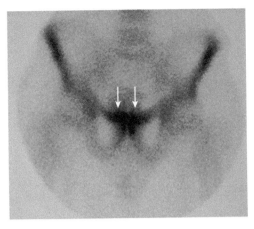

Fig. 8.9 Isotope bone scan of a 27-year-old soccer player with osteitis pubis shows concentration of radiotracer activity at the symphysis pubis with increased marginal osteoblastic activity *(arrows)*. (From MacMahon PJ, Hogan BA, Shelly MJ, et al. Imaging of groin pain. *Magn Reson Imaging Clin N Am.* 2009;17:655−666.)

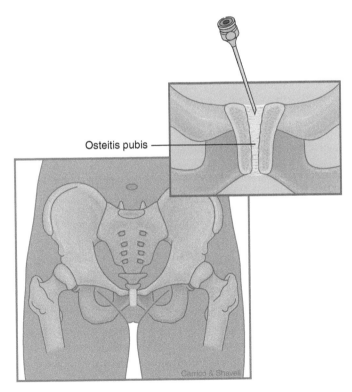

Osteitis pubis

Fig. 8.10 Proper needle placement for injection of osteitis pubis. (From Waldman SD. *Atlas of Pain Management Injection Techniques.* 4th ed. St Louis: Elsevier; 2017: Fig. 126-4.)

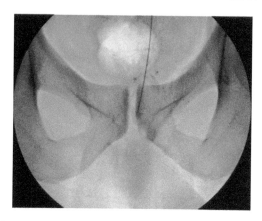

Fig. 8.11 Fluoroscopic needle placement for injection of the symphysis pubis. (From Waldman SD. *Atlas of Pain Management Injection Techniques*. 4th ed. St Louis: Elsevier; 2017: Fig. 126-5.)

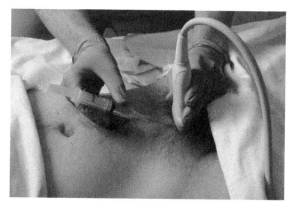

Fig. 8.12 Proper needle placement for an ultrasound-guided out-of-plane injection for osteitis pubis. (Courtesy Steven D. Waldman, MD.)

identified by palpation, and the overlying skin is prepared with antiseptic solution. A syringe containing 2 mL of 0.25% preservative-free bupivacaine and 40 mg methylprednisolone is attached to a 3.5-inch, 25-gauge needle. The needle is advanced very slowly through the previously identified point at a right angle to the skin, directly toward the center of the symphysis pubis (see Fig. 8.10). Once the needle impinges on the fibroelastic cartilage of the joint, it is withdrawn slightly out of the joint. After careful aspiration for blood and if no paresthesia is present, the contents of the syringe are gently injected. Resistance to injection should be minimal. The use of fluoroscopic or ultrasound needle guidance will improve the accuracy of needle placement and decrease the incidence of needle-related complications (Figs. 8.11 and 8.12). This technique can also be used for prolotherapy of the pubic symphysis and for obtaining cultures of the joint.

Physical modalities, including local heat and gentle stretching exercises, should be introduced several days after the patient undergoes injection. Vigorous exercises should be avoided because they will exacerbate patient symptoms. Simple analgesics, NSAIDs, and antimyotonic agents such as tizanidine may be used concurrently with this injection technique.

HIGH-YIELD TAKEAWAYS

- The patient's symptomatology began after a cesarean section complicated by persistent urinary tract infections.
- The patient's pain is localized to the symphysis pubis.
- The patient has a waddling gait, which is highly suggestive of osteitis pubis.
- The patient is afebrile, making an acute infectious etiology (e.g., postoperative infection or urosepsis) unlikely.
- The lower extremity neurologic examination is within normal limits, making a central spinal or lumbar plexus lesion much less likely.
- The X-ray of the symphysis pubis demonstrates characteristic findings, as does the MRI.

Suggested Readings

Budak MJ, Oliver TB. There's a hole in my symphysis—a review of disorders causing widening, erosion, and destruction of the symphysis pubis. *Clin Radiol.* 2013;68 (2):173–180.

Elshout PJ, Verleyen P, Putzeys G. Osteitis pubis after TURP: a rare complication difficult to recognize. *Urol Case Rep.* 2016;4:55–58.

Glasser JG. Case report: osteitis/osteomyelitis pubis simulating acute appendicitis. *Int J Surg Case Rep.* 2018;53:269–272.

Waldman SD. Injection Technique for Osteitis Pubis. In: *Atlas of Pain Management Injection Techniques.* 4th ed. Philadelphia: Elsevier; 2017:458–461.

Waldman SD. Osteitis Pubis. In: *Atlas of Common Pain Syndromes.* 4th ed. Philadelphia: Elsevier; 2017:311–314.

Waldman SD. Osteitis Pubis. In: *Pain Review.* 2nd ed. Philadelphia: Elsevier; 2017: 296–297.

Waldman SD. Osteitis Pubis and Other Abnormalities of the Pubic Symphysis. In: *Waldman's Comprehensive Atlas of Diagnostic Ultrasound of Painful Conditions.* Philadelphia: Kluwer Wolters; 2016:640–646.

Waldman SD, Campbell RSD. Anatomy: Special Imaging Considerations of the Sacroiliac Joint and Pelvis. In: *Imaging of Pain.* Philadelphia: Elsevier; 2011:192–196.

Waldman SD, Campbell RSD. Osteitis Pubis. In: *Imaging of Pain.* Philadelphia: Elsevier; 2011:207–208.

Avi Rudin

A 68-Year-Old Male With Anterior Thigh and Medial Calf Pain and Difficulty Walking Up Stairs

- Learn the common causes of lower extremity numbness.
- Develop an understanding of the anatomy of the femoral nerve.
- Develop an understanding of the unique relationship of the femoral nerve to the inguinal ligament.
- Develop an understanding of the unique relationship of the femoral nerve to the femoral artery and vein.
- Develop an understanding of the causes of femoral neuropathy.
- Develop an understanding of the differential diagnosis of lower extremity pain and numbness.
- Learn the clinical presentation of femoral neuropathy.
- Learn the dermatomes of the lower extremity.
- Learn how to use physical examination to identify femoral neuropathy.
- Develop an understanding of the treatment options for femoral neuropathy.

Avi Rudin

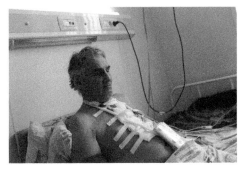

Avi Rudin is a 68-year-old violinist with the chief complaint of, "Ever since my cardiac cath, I've had pain and numbness in my left leg." Avi stated that a couple of months ago, he was shoveling snow off his front walk when he began having crushing chest pain and lightheadedness. He called 911 and was rushed to the emergency room. He was seen by a cardiologist who diagnosed an ST-elevation myocardial infarction (STEMI) and suggested a cardiac catherization with probable angioplasty and coronary artery stent. Avi said that he doesn't remember much about the cardiac catherization, but clearly remembers feeling an electric shock that went down his leg when the doctor put the needle into his groin. Avi went on to say that the cath "didn't work" and he had to have a four-vessel cardiac bypass. The first thing he remembered when he woke up after his surgery was this burning pain that ran from his groin into the front of his left leg and then down into his medial calf. He said his chest incision hurt, but it was the leg pain that really bothered him. Avi said that his doctor told him not to worry, that it was just a little nerve irritation from the cardiac cath and it would get better with time, but it never did.

I asked Avi if he had experienced any numbness or weakness in his legs and he replied, "Doc, it's funny that you asked because over the last couple of weeks, I have really had a lot of trouble walking up stairs or lifting my leg up to put on my socks." "Both legs?" I asked, and he said "No, just the left." I asked Avi what he had tried to make it better and he said that massaging his thigh seemed to help a little, but the pain pills he had for after his heart surgery just made him sick to his stomach, so he quit taking them.

He also volunteered that he had stopped wearing pajama bottoms to bed because the skin over the painful area was so sensitive, "kind of like a sunburn," Avi reported. "Also, Tylenol PM seems to help some, at least with sleep."

I asked Avi to show me where the pain was and he pointed to his left anterior thigh and then reached down and patted his medial calf. I asked Avi about any fever, chills or other constitutional symptoms such as weight loss, night sweats, etc., and he shook his head no. He denied any further chest pain, but said the pain often woke him up at night.

On physical examination, Avi was afebrile. His respirations were 18, his pulse was 74 and regular, and his blood pressure was 122/78. Avi's head, eyes, ears, nose, throat (HEENT) exam was normal, as was his thyroid exam. Auscultation of his carotids revealed no bruits, and the pulses in all four extremities were normal. He had a regular rhythm without abnormal beats. His cardiac exam was otherwise unremarkable. There was a well-healed median sternotomy scar without defect or evidence of infection. His abdominal examination revealed no abnormal mass or organomegaly. There was no peripheral edema. His low back examination was unremarkable. There was no costovertebral angle (CVA) tenderness. Visual inspection of the left lower extremity was unremarkable. There was no rubor or color, but there was mild allodynia in the distribution of the femoral nerve on the left. There was no obvious infection. There was no femoral bruit. Examination of his right lower extremity revealed a well-healed scar from harvest of his saphenous vein for his coronary artery grafts.

A careful neurologic examination of both lower extremities revealed decreased sensation in the distribution of the left femoral nerve and marked weakness of the left quadriceps muscle (Fig. 9.1). His femoral stretch test on the left was markedly positive (Fig. 9.2). The right lower extremity neurologic examination was completely normal, other than subtle numbness in the distribution of his saphenous nerve, presumably from the vein harvest. Deep tendon reflexes were normal except for a decreased knee jerk on the left. There was a positive Tinel sign over the left femoral nerve.

Key Clinical Points—What's Important and What's Not

THE HISTORY

- A history of the onset of anterior thigh and medial calf pain immediately following a cardiac catherization
- Difficulty walking up stairs
- Difficulty fully extending the left leg
- Pain has a sunburn like quality
- No symptoms in the right lower extremity
- No fever or chills
- History of recent coronary artery bypass surgery

THE PHYSICAL EXAMINATION

- The patient is afebrile
- Marked weakness of the quadriceps muscle on the left
- Numbness in the distribution of the femoral nerve on the left (see Fig. 9.1)
- Positive femoral stretch test (see Fig. 9.2)
- Positive Tinel sign over the femoral nerve on the left
- Allodynia in the distribution of the left femoral nerve

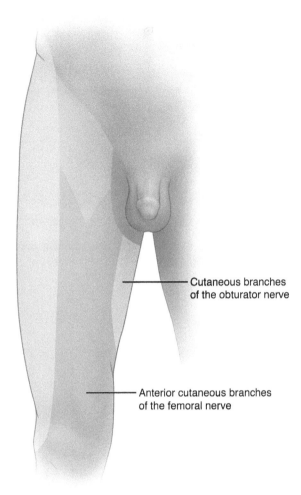

Cutaneous branches
of the obturator nerve

Anterior cutaneous branches
of the femoral nerve

Fig. 9.1 The sensory distribution of the femoral nerve. (From Waldman SD. *Atlas of Pain Management Injection Techniques*. 4th ed. St Louis: Elsevier; 2017: Fig. 110-2.)

- No motor deficit in the right lower extremity
- Deep tendon reflexes within normal limits bilaterally except for a decreased knee jerk on the left

OTHER FINDINGS OF NOTE

- Normal HEENT examination
- Normal cardiovascular examination
- Normal pulmonary examination
- Normal abdominal examination

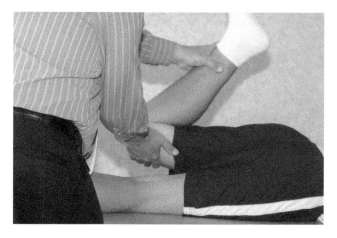

Fig. 9.2   The femoral stretch test. Have the patient lie prone. Passively flex the knee as far as it goes. In a positive test, the patient should feel pain in the ipsilateral anterior thigh (i.e., the distribution of the femoral nerve). Also, pain may be exacerbated on hip extension. (From Waldman SD. *Physical Diagnosis of Pain: An Atlas of Signs and Symptoms.* 3rd ed. St Louis: Elsevier; 2016: Fig. 170-1.)

- No peripheral edema
- No carotid or femoral bruits

 ## What Tests Would You Like to Order?

The following tests were ordered:
- Ultrasound of the left femoral nerve at the level of the inguinal ligament
- Electromyography (EMG) and nerve conduction velocity testing of the left femoral nerve

TEST RESULTS

Ultrasound examination of the femoral nerve at the level of the femoral triangle reveals no obvious tumor or mass compressing the femoral nerve (Fig. 9.3). EMG and nerve conduction velocity testing revealed slowing of femoral nerve conduction across the femoral triangle. Needle examination reveals marked denervation of the quadriceps muscle

 ## Clinical Correlation—Putting It All Together

What is the diagnosis?
- Femoral neuropathy secondary to needle-induced trauma during a cardiac catherization

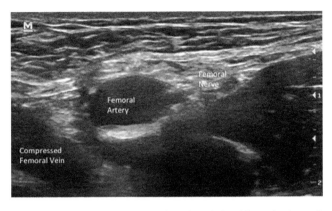

Fig. 9.3 Ultrasound image of the femoral nerve. Note the relationship to the femoral artery and vein, which has been compressed with the ultrasound transducer to facilitate identification. (Courtesy Steven Waldman, MD.)

The Science Behind the Diagnosis

ANATOMY

The largest branch of the lumbar plexus, the femoral nerve is derived from the posterior branches of the L2, L3, and L4 nerve roots. The nerve fibers enter the psoas muscle, where they fuse together within the muscle body and then descend laterally between the psoas and iliacus muscles. The femoral nerve provides motor innervation to the iliacus muscle as it descends toward the iliac fossa. The nerve then passes just lateral to the femoral artery, lying on top of the ilacus muscle and beneath the fascia iliaca as it travels beneath the inguinal ligament with the artery, vein, and nerve enclosed in the femoral sheath (Figs. 9.4 and 9.5). It is at this point that the nerve can consistently be identified with ultrasound scanning and is amenable to ultrasound-guided nerve block. The femoral nerve provides motor innervation to the sartorius, quadriceps femoris, and pectineus muscles and provides sensory fibers to the knee joint as well as the skin overlying the anterior thigh (Fig. 9.6; see Fig. 9.1).

CLINICAL SYNDROME

The proximity of the femoral nerve, artery, and vein to each other make them subject to compromise from traumatic injury, hematoma, abnormal mass, and tumors. The femoral nerve is subject to the development of neuropathy from a variety of causes, including compression, iatrogenic trauma, metabolic abnormalities, vasculitis, ischemia, and most notably, diabetes mellitus. The clinical findings of femoral neuropathy include weakness of the quadriceps femoris and occasionally the iliacus muscle, diminished or absent knee jerk, and sensory loss

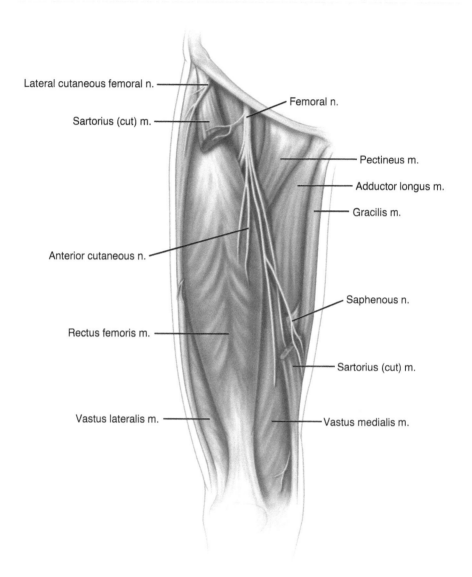

Lateral cutaneous femoral n.

Sartorius (cut) m.

Femoral n.

Pectineus m.

Adductor longus m.

Gracilis m.

Anterior cutaneous n.

Saphenous n.

Rectus femoris m.

Sartorius (cut) m.

Vastus lateralis m.

Vastus medialis m.

Fig. 9.4 Anatomy of the femoral nerve. *m.*, Muscle; *n.*, nerve. (From Waldman SD. *Atlas of Pain Management Injection Techniques*. 4th ed. St Louis: Elsevier; 2017: Fig. 110-1.)

over the anteromedial aspect of the thigh and medial aspect of the lower leg. Spontaneous retroperitoneal hematomas within the psoas—iliacus groove in anticoagulated patients can severely compress the femoral nerve (Fig. 9.7). The femoral nerve, artery, and vein also can be compressed by tumor, lymphadenopathy, and abscess. The neurovascular bundle is subject to traumatic injury from penetrating injuries; hip fracture; iatrogenic injuries during abdominal, pelvic,

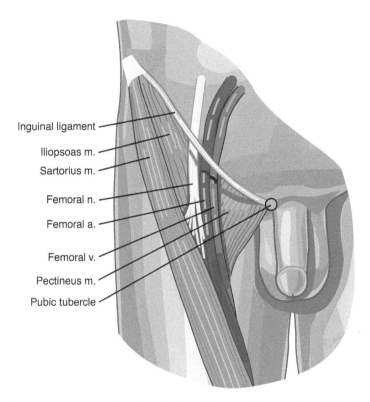

Fig. 9.5 The femoral nerve is just lateral to the femoral artery as it passes beneath the inguinal ligament and is enclosed within the femoral sheath along with the femoral artery and vein. *a.,* Artery; *m.,* muscle; *n.,* nerve: *v.,* vein. (From Waldman SD. *Atlas of Pain Management Injection Techniques.* 4th ed. St Louis: Elsevier; 2017: Fig. 110-3.)

groin, and hip surgery; and injuries from needle-induced trauma during femoral arterial cannulation for cardiac catherization.

SIGNS AND SYMPTOMS

The patient with femoral neuropathy will present with pain that radiates into the anterior thigh and medial calf. This pain may be paresthetic or burning in character. The intensity is moderate to severe. Weakness of the quadriceps muscle can be quite marked, making walking upstairs or fully extending the leg difficult (Fig. 9.8). If femoral nerve compromise persists, over time atrophy of the quadriceps may occur, especially in diabetic patients (Fig. 9.9). Patients with femoral neuropathy may complain of a sunburned feeling over the anterior thigh. The patient may also complain that the knee feels like it is giving way.

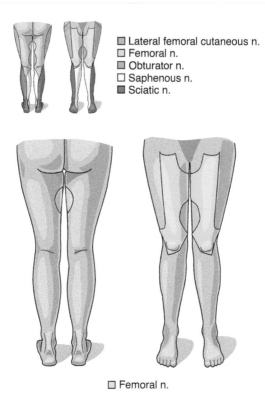

☐ Lateral femoral cutaneous n.
☐ Femoral n.
☐ Obturator n.
☐ Saphenous n.
■ Sciatic n.

☐ Femoral n.

Fig. 9.6 Sensory distribution of the femoral nerve. *n.*, Nerve. (From Waldman SD. *Atlas of Pain Management Injection Techniques*. 4th ed. St Louis: Elsevier; 2017: Fig. 110-4.)

TESTING

EMG can distinguish femoral nerve compromise from lumbar plexopathy and lumbar radiculopathy. Plain radiographs of the hip and pelvis are indicated in all patients who present with femoral neuralgia to rule out occult bony pathology. Based on the patient's clinical presentation, additional testing may be warranted, including a complete blood count, uric acid level, erythrocyte sedimentation rate, and antinuclear antibody testing. Magnetic resonance imaging (MRI) of the lumbar spine and lumbar plexus and retroperitoneum is indicated if herniated disc, tumor, or hematoma is suspected. Ultrasonography and Doppler evaluation of the femoral artery and nerve can help identify thrombus, embolus, occlusion by hematoma, tumor, abscess, foreign bodies (e.g., bullet fragments), clot, and arteriosclerotic plaque (see Fig. 9.3). Injection of the femoral nerve with local anesthetic may serve as both a diagnostic and a therapeutic maneuver (Fig. 9.10).

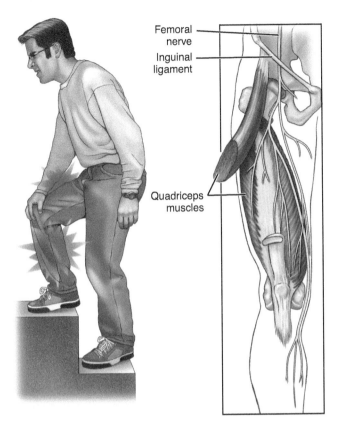

Femoral
nerve

Inguinal
ligament

Quadriceps
muscles

Fig. 9.7 Patients with femoral neuropathy present with pain that radiates into the anterior thigh and medial calf with associated weakness of the quadriceps muscle. (From Waldman SD. *Atlas of Uncommon Pain Syndromes*. 4th ed. Philadelphia: Saunders; 2020: Fig. 105.1.)

DIFFERENTIAL DIAGNOSIS

Femoral neuropathy is often misdiagnosed as lumbar radiculopathy, trochanteric bursitis, meralgia paresthetica, or primary hip pathology. Radiographs of the hip and electromyography can distinguish femoral neuropathy from radiculopathy or pain emanating from the hip. In addition, most patients suffering from lumbar radiculopathy have back pain associated with reflex, motor, and sensory changes, whereas patients with femoral neuropathy have no back pain and no motor or reflex changes; the sensory changes of femoral neuropathy are limited to the distribution of the femoral nerve and should not extend below the knee. It should be remembered that lumbar radiculopathy and femoral nerve entrapment may coexist as the "double-crush" syndrome. Occasionally, diabetic femoral neuropathy produces anterior thigh pain, which may confuse the diagnosis.

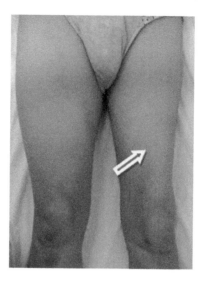

Fig. 9.8 Amyotrophy of the left quadriceps femoris. (From Jellad A, Boudokhane S, Ezzine S, et al. Femoral neuropathy caused by compressive iliopsoas hydatid cyst: a case report and review of the literature. *Joint Bone Spine.* 2010;77:371–372.)

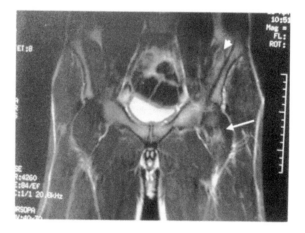

Fig. 9.9 T2-weighted coronal magnetic resonance imaging showing the hematoma as an area of increased signal intensity in the muscle belly *(arrowhead)*. Fascial edema/hemorrhage is depicted as linear hyperintensity. An ill-defined area of high signal intensity can be seen at the distal myotendinous junction of the left psoas–iliacus complex, indicating a partial injury *(arrow)*. (From Seijo-Martínez M, Castro del Río M, Fontoira E, et al. Acute femoral neuropathy secondary to an iliacus muscle hematoma. *J Neurol Sci.* 2003;209:119–122.)

TREATMENT

Mild cases of femoral neuropathy will usually respond to conservative therapy, and surgery should be reserved for more severe cases. Initial treatment of

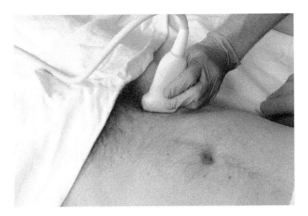

Fig. 9.10 Ultrasound-guided injection of the femoral nerve with local anesthetic may serve as both a diagnostic and a therapeutic maneuver. (Courtesy Steven Waldman, MD.)

femoral neuropathy should consist of treatment with simple analgesics, nonsteroidal antiinflammatory agents, or cyclooxygenase-2 inhibitors. If diabetes is thought to be the etiology of the patient's femoral neuropathy, tight control of blood sugars is mandatory. Avoidance of repetitive activities thought to be responsible for the exacerbation of femoral neuropathy (e.g., repetitive hip extension and flexion) will also help ameliorate patient symptoms. If the patient fails to respond to these conservative measures, a next reasonable step is injection of the femoral nerve with a local anesthetic and steroid. The use of gabapentin and pregabalin may help reduce the parethesias associated with femoral neuropathy.

HIGH-YIELD TAKEAWAYS

- The patient is afebrile, making an acute infectious etiology unlikely.
- The patient's symptomatology is thought to be the result of trauma to the femoral nerve during femoral artery catherization.
- Physical examination and testing should be focused on identification of other pathologic processes that may mimic the clinical diagnosis of femoral neuropathy.
- The patient exhibits the neurologic and physical examination findings that are highly suggestive of femoral neuropathy.
- The patient's symptoms are unilateral.
- EMG and nerve conduction velocity testing will help delineate the location and degree of nerve compromise if femoral nerve compression is suspected.
- Ultrasound imaging of the femoral nerve may help identify less common causes of compression of the nerve (e.g., tumor, lipoma, or neural tumors).

Suggested Readings

Craig A. Entrapment neuropathies of the lower extremity. *PM&R*. 2013;5(5):S31—S40.

Fridman V, David WS. Electrodiagnostic evaluation of lower extremity mononeuro-pathies. *Neurol Clin*. 2012;30(2):505—528.

Ganu S, Mehta Y. Femoral compressive neuropathy from iliopsoas haematoma compli-cating dengue hemorrhagic fever. *Asian Pac J Trop Med*. 2013;6(5):419—420.

Kothari G, Sinha A. Femoral neuropathy caused by psoas schwannoma: a case report. *PM&R*. 2013;5(9):S292—S293.

Leung P, Kudrna JC. Growth of an intrapelvic pseudotumor associated with a metal-on-metal total hip arthroplasty after revision arthroplasty causing a femoral nerve neuropathy. *Arthroplast*. 2016;2(3):105—109.

Waldman SD. Abnormalities of the femoral nerve, artery, and vein. In: *Comprehensive Atlas of Diagnosis Ultrasound of Painful Conditions*. Philadelphia: Wolters Kluwer; 2016:622—628.

Waldman SD. Femoral neuropathy. In: *Atlas of Uncommon Pain Syndromes*. 4th ed. Philadelphia: Elsevier; 2020:388—394.

Mario Berbiglia

A 72-Year-Old Male With Medial Thigh Pain Following a Total Hip Arthroplasty

LEARNING OBJECTIVES

- Learn the common causes of lower extremity numbness.
- Develop an understanding of the unique relationship of the obturator nerve to the inguinal ligaments.
- Develop an understanding of the anatomy of the obturator nerve.
- Develop an understanding of the causes of obturator neuralgia.
- Develop an understanding of the differential diagnosis of obturator neuralgia.
- Learn the clinical presentation of obturator neuralgia.
- Learn the dermatomes of the lower extremity.
- Learn how to use physical examination to identify obturator neuralgia.
- Develop an understanding of the treatment options for obturator neuralgia.

Mario Berbiglia

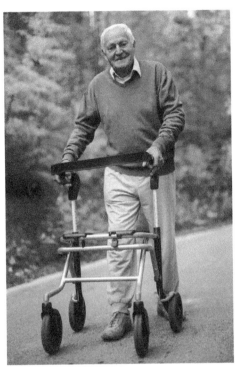

Mario Berbiglia is a 72-year-old restaurant owner with the chief complaint of, "I'm having sharp pain in my inner thigh since that damn hip replacement." Mario shook his head and said, "I should have never had it done, but I wanted to keep working and I thought it would help." Mario went on to state that he had pain in his left inner thigh before he even got up to the side of the bed following his total hip arthroplasty. His orthopedic surgeon said that some pain after surgery was to be expected, but even when the postoperative pain went away, the thigh pain continued. Mario said that he was trying to do everything his physical therapist told him to do, but "the pain is really limiting my recovery, and now my left leg feels unsteady." When he went back for his 8-week follow-up with the orthopedic surgeon, he felt like the surgeon couldn't have cared less and finally told him that he would just have to learn to live with the pain, as the surgery was a complete success. Mario said, "Yeah, the surgery was a complete success, but the patient died! Doc, I am really getting discouraged. My kids are trying to keep the restaurant going, but my customers expect me to be there to greet them like I've been doing for the past 35 years. Villa Capri without Mario is like spaghetti without meatballs. I really need to get back to my customers, but I don't want them to see me with this damn walker."

I asked Mario to show me where the pain was, and he rubbed his left inner thigh (Fig. 10.1). "Doc, it's right here. There is always a deep ache and when I try to walk, I get electric shocks into the area. It's really discouraging. What the hell did that doctor do to me? I should have never gone under the knife! I knew better." I asked Mario about any fever, chills, or other constitutional symptoms such as weight loss, night sweats, etc., and he shook his head no. He also denied bowel or bladder symptomatology. He denied any antecedent lower extremity trauma, but noted that the pain woke him up "about 50 times a night" and that it was making him cranky.

He then asked, "Doc, tell me the truth. What do you think this guy did to me?" I clapped Mario on the shoulder and said that I would do my best to

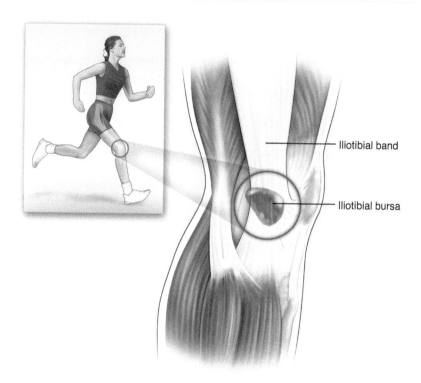

Fig. 10.1 Patients with obturator neuralgia typically have pain that radiates into the medial thigh and does not extend below the knee. (From Waldman SD. *Atlas of Uncommon Pain Syndromes*. 4th ed. Philadelphia: Saunders; 2020: Fig. 107.1.)

figure out what was going on and together we would come up with a plan to make it better.

On physical examination, Mario was afebrile. His respirations were 18, his pulse was 74 and regular, and his blood pressure was 132/78. His head, eyes, ears, nose, throat (HEENT) exam was normal, as was his cardiopulmonary examination. His thyroid was normal. His abdominal examination revealed no abnormal mass or organomegaly. There was no costovertebral angle (CVA) tenderness. There was no peripheral edema. His low back examination was unremarkable. Visual inspection of the left lower extremity was unremarkable other than his well-healed hip surgery scar. There was no obvious infection. There was no rubor or color in the painful area, and there was no evidence of abnormal mass or hernia. Rectal and testicular examinations were normal, other than a small external hemorrhoid. I asked Mario to walk down the hall. He did pretty well getting up with the help of his walker, but his gait was antalgic as he slowly walked down the hall. I also noted that Mario's left foot was externally rotated (see accompanying photo on page 123).

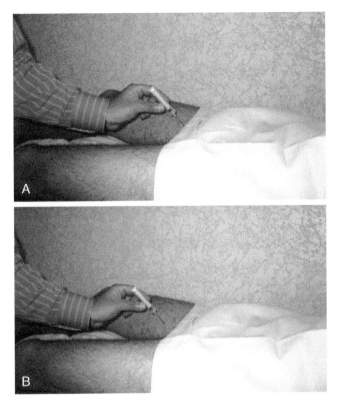

Fig. 10.2 (A, B) The numb medial thigh sign for obturator nerve entrapment. (From Waldman SD. *Physical Diagnosis of Pain: An Atlas of Signs and Symptoms*. 3rd ed. St Louis: Elsevier; 2016: Fig. 168-2.)

A careful neurologic examination of both lower extremities revealed a slight decrease in sensation in the distribution of the left obturator nerve, but no sensory abnormalities below the knee were identified. A numb medial thigh sign was present (Fig. 10.2). There was allodynia in the distribution of the obturator nerve on the left. His left lower extremity motor exam revealed moderate weakness of the hip adductors, which could account for that "unsteady feeling." His right lower extremity neurologic examination was completely normal. Deep tendon reflexes were normal throughout the upper extremity, knee jerks were physiologic, and ankle jerks were trace but symmetrical bilaterally.

Key Clinical Points—What's Important and What's Not

THE HISTORY

- A history of the onset of medial thigh pain following a total hip arthroplasty
- A sense that the left lower extremity is "unsteady"

- Pain symptomatology limiting physical therapy
- Pain is characterized as a deep pain with electric shocklike pain into the medial thigh when ambulating
- No symptoms in the right lower extremity
- No fever or chills
- No bowel or bladder symptomatology

THE PHYSICAL EXAMINATION

- The patient is afebrile
- Decreased sensation in the distribution of the left obturator nerve
- No sensory deficit below the knee on the left
- Allodynia in the distribution of the left obturator nerve
- Weakness of the hip adductors on the left
- No motor deficit in the right lower extremity
- Deep tendon reflexes are physiologic
- Antalgic gait

OTHER FINDINGS OF NOTE

- Normal HEENT examination
- Normal cardiovascular examination
- Normal pulmonary examination
- Normal abdominal examination
- No abnormal mass or hernia noted
- No peripheral edema

 What Tests Would You Like to Order?

The following tests were ordered:
- X-ray of the left hip
- Computed tomography (CT) of the left hip
- Electromyography (EMG) and nerve conduction velocity testing of the left obturator nerve

TEST RESULTS

Anteroposterior radiograph of the left hip reveals extrapelvic cement extrusion from the total hip arthroplasty (Fig. 10.3). CT of the left hip reveals intrapelvic extrusion of bone cement (Fig. 10.4). EMG and nerve conduction velocity testing revealed slowing of obturator nerve conduction and denervation of the hip adductors on the left.

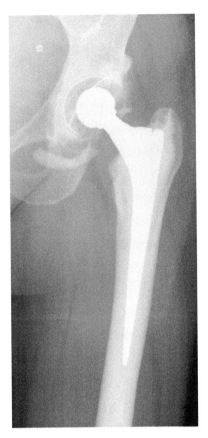

Fig. 10.3 Anteroposterior radiograph of the left hip demonstrating extrapelvic cement extrusion from the total hip arthroplasty. (From Mahadevan D, Challand C, Keenan J. Cement extrusion during hip arthroplasty causing pain and obturator nerve impingement. *J Arthroplasty*. 2009;24[1]:158.e1−158.e3 [Fig. 1].)

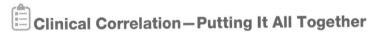 **Clinical Correlation—Putting It All Together**

What is the diagnosis?
- Obturator neuralgia

The Science Behind the Diagnosis

ANATOMY

The obturator nerve is derived from the posterior branches of the L2, L3, and L4 nerve roots (Fig. 10.5). The nerve fibers enter the psoas muscle, where they fuse together within the muscle body and leave the medial border of the psoas at the

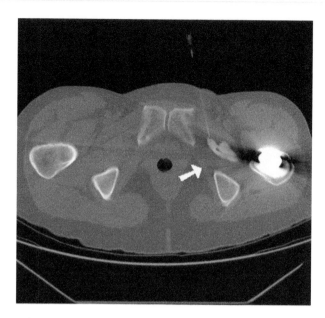

Fig. 10.4 Computed tomography scan showing intrapelvic cement fragment. Arrow showing marked atrophy of thigh adductor compartment. (From Mahadevan D, Challand C, Keenan J. Cement extrusion during hip arthroplasty causing pain and obturator nerve impingement. *J Arthroplasty*. 2009;24[1]: 158.e1–158.e3 [Fig. 2].)

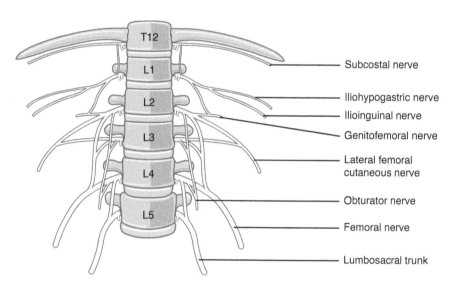

Fig. 10.5 The obturator nerve provides most of the innervation to the hip joint. It is derived from the posterior divisions of the L2, L3, and L4 nerves of the lumbar plexus. (From Waldman SD. *Atlas of Interventional Pain Management*. 4th ed. Philadelphia: Saunders; 2015: Fig. 126-2.)

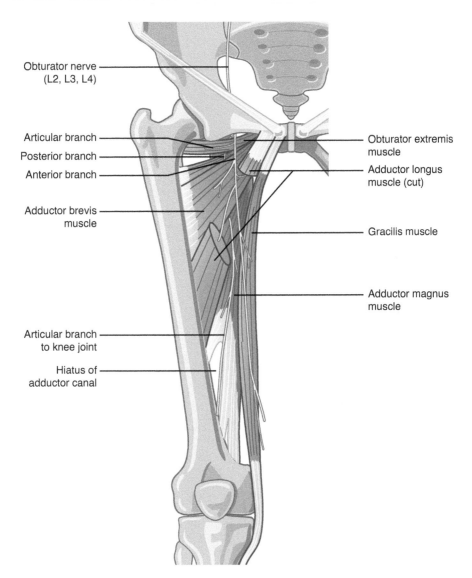

Obturator nerve
(L2, L3, L4)

Articular branch

Posterior branch

Anterior branch

Adductor brevis
muscle

Articular branch
to knee joint

Hiatus of
adductor canal

Obturator extremis
muscle

Adductor longus
muscle (cut)

Gracilis muscle

Adductor magnus
muscle

Fig. 10.6 Anatomy of the obturator nerve. (From Waldman SD. *Atlas of Interventional Pain Management*. 4th ed. Philadelphia: Saunders; 2015: Fig. 126-3.)

brim of the pelvis (Fig. 10.6). The nerve passes behind the common iliac arteries to run adjacent to the lateral wall of the pelvis, where it joins the obturator artery and vein. Along with the obturator artery and vein, the obturator nerve enters the obturator canal to pass into the proximal thigh. At this point, the nerve divides into an anterior branch, which provides sensory innervation to the hip joint, motor branches to the superficial hip adductors, a cutaneous branch to the

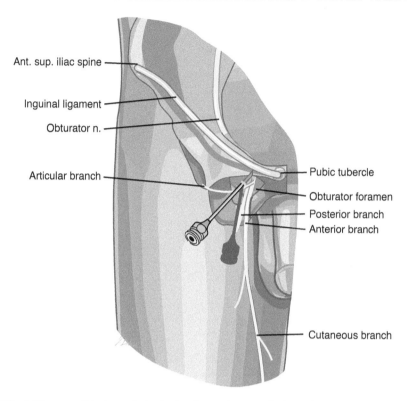

Fig. 10.7 A 22-gauge, 3-inch needle is slowly advanced perpendicular to the skin until the needle is felt to impinge on the superior pubic ramus. *Ant.*, Anterior; *n.*, nerve; *sup.*, superior. (From Waldman SD. *Atlas of Interventional Pain Management.* 4th ed. Philadelphia: Saunders; 2015: Fig. 126-6.)

medial aspect of the distal thigh, a posterior branch, which provides motor innervation to the deep hip adductors, and an articular branch to the posterior knee joint (Figs. 10.7 and 10.8).

CLINICAL SYNDROME

The obturator nerve is subject to compression, entrapment, and trauma from the point where it fuses together within the psoas muscle and travels inferiorly along with the obturator artery and vein to enter the obturator canal, as well as along its inferior path as it passes between the adductor brevis and longus muscles. The nerve may be compressed and entrapped by retroperitoneal and pelvic cysts, tumors, hematoma, endometriosis, and callus formation from healing pelvic fractures as well as by implantable mesh and tapes used for surgical correction of urinary incontinence and uterine prolapse (Figs. 10.9 and 10.10). The nerve may be injured by penetrating

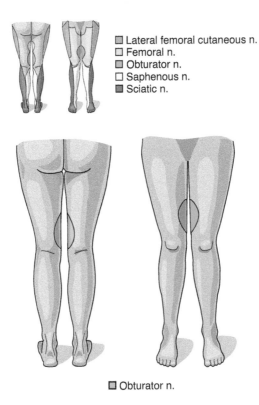

☐ Lateral femoral cutaneous n.
☐ Femoral n.
☐ Obturator n.
☐ Saphenous n.
■ Sciatic n.

☐ Obturator n.

Fig. 10.8 Sensory distribution of the obturator nerve. *n.*, Nerve. (From Waldman SD. *Atlas of Interventional Pain Management.* 4th ed. Philadelphia: Saunders; 2015: Fig. 126-5.)

injuries as well as from pelvic fractures, tumor, crush injuries, midforceps deliveries, and surgical misadventures during groin, pelvic, and medial thigh surgeries.

SIGNS AND SYMPTOMS

Patients with significant obturator neuropathy lose the ability to abduct and externally rotate the hip. The patient will exhibit a typical gait abnormality that consists of an externally rotated foot, as shown in the chapter opening photo. Wasting of the adductor muscles of the thigh and numbness of the distal medial thigh may also be identified. Deep, aching groin pain is often present, which is often centered on the attachment of the adductor muscles to the pubic bone. Exercise will often exacerbate the pain and may cause paresthesias to radiate into the distribution of the anterior division of the obturator nerve on the medial thigh. These symptoms may often be reproduced by active external rotation of the hip against resistance.

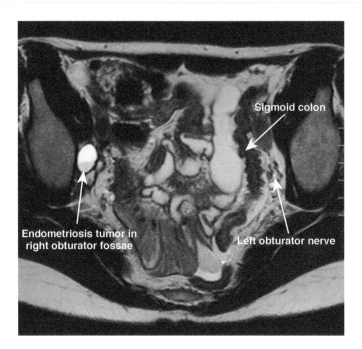

Fig. 10.9 Transverse magnetic resonance image of the pelvis, with entrapment of the obturator nerve on the right side. (From Langebrekke A, Qvigstad E. Endometriosis entrapment of the obturator nerve after previous cervical cancer surgery. *Fertil Steril.* 2009;91:622–623.)

TESTING

EMG can help identify the exact source of neurologic dysfunction and clarify the differential diagnosis, and should be the starting point of the evaluation of all patients thought to have obturator neuralgia. Plain radiographs of the spine, hip, pelvis, and proximal femur are indicated in all patients with obturator neuralgia to rule out occult bony pathology. Based on the patient's clinical presentation, additional tests, including complete blood cell count, uric acid level, erythrocyte sedimentation rate, and antinuclear antibody testing, may be indicated. Magnetic resonance imaging (MRI) of the spine, pelvis, and proximal lower extremity is indicated if tumor, hematoma, or other abnormality is suspected (see Fig. 10.9). CT scanning may be useful to identify abnormalities in patients in whom implants may preclude the use of MRI (see Fig. 10.4). Ultrasound imaging may also provide useful information regarding the status of the nerve (Fig. 10.11). Injection of the obturator nerve with a local anesthetic and steroid serves as a diagnostic and therapeutic maneuver. Fluoroscopic or ultrasound guidance may improve the accuracy of needle placement (Fig. 10.12).

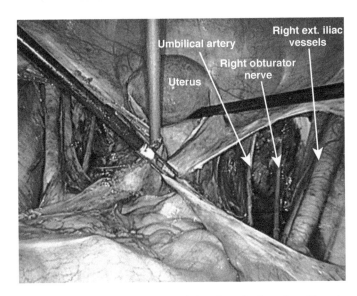

Fig. 10.10   Overview of the pelvis after laparoscopic lymph node dissection. (From Langebrekke A, Qvigstad E. Endometriosis entrapment of the obturator nerve after previous cervical cancer surgery. *Fertil Steril.* 2009;91:622–623.)

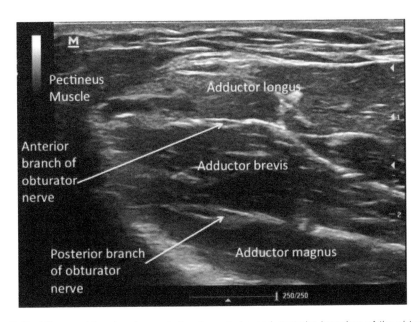

Fig. 10.11   Ultrasound imaging demonstrating the anterior and posterior branches of the obturator nerve. (Courtesy Steven D. Waldman, MD.)

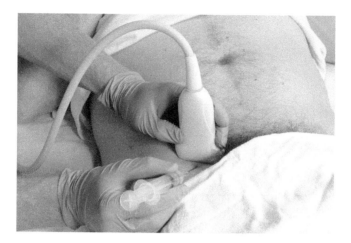

Fig. 10.12 When the adductor muscles and the anterior and posterior branches of the obturator nerve have been identified, the skin is prepared with anesthetic solution and a 22-gauge, 1.5-inch needle is introduced at the inferior border of the ultrasound transducer and advanced using an out-of-plane approach, with the trajectory adjusted under real-time ultrasound guidance so that the needle passes through the adductor longus muscle and the needle tip rests in the fascial cleft between the adductor longus and brevis muscles in proximity to the anterior branch of the obturator nerve. After satisfactory injection of the anterior branch, the needle is then withdrawn and redirected through both the adductor longus and the brevis muscles until the needle tip rests in the fascial cleft between the adductor brevis and magnus muscles in proximity to the posterior branch of the obturator nerve. After careful aspiration, the posterior branch is injected. (From Waldman SD. *Atlas of Interventional Pain Management.* 4th ed. Philadelphia: Saunders; 2015: Fig. 126-17.)

DIFFERENTIAL DIAGNOSIS

It is sometimes difficult to separate obturator neuralgia from a lumbar plexopathy or radiculopathy on purely clinical grounds, and EMG is strongly recommended. EMG and nerve conduction testing also help rule out the presence of peripheral neuropathy. Intrapelvic or retroperitoneal tumor or hematoma may compress the lumbar plexus and mimic the clinical presentation of obturator neuralgia.

TREATMENT

Mild cases of obturator neuralgia usually respond to conservative therapy, and surgery should be reserved for more severe cases. Initial treatment of obturator neuralgia should consist of treatment with simple analgesics, nonsteroidal antiinflammatory drugs, or cyclooxygenase-2 inhibitors and avoidance of repetitive activities that exacerbate the symptoms. If diabetes is thought to be the cause of the patient's obturator neuralgia, tight control of blood glucose levels is mandatory. Avoidance of repetitive activities thought to be responsible for the exacerbation of obturator neuralgia also helps ameliorate the symptoms. The use of gabapentin or a tricyclic antidepressant such as nortriptyline as an adjuvant analgesic also may help ameliorate the symptoms of obturator neuralgia. If the patient fails to respond to these conservative measures, a reasonable next step is injection of the obturator nerve with a local anesthetic and steroid. Ultrasound imaging may improve the accuracy of needle placement and decrease the incidence of needle-related complications.

HIGH-YIELD TAKEAWAYS

- The patient is afebrile, making an acute infectious etiology unlikely.
- The patient's symptomatology is thought to be the result of compression of the left obturator nerve by extruded bone cement from a total hip arthroplasty.
- Physical examination and testing should be focused on identification of other pathologic processes that may mimic the clinical diagnosis of obturator neuralgia.
- The patient exhibits the neurologic and physical examination findings that are highly suggestive of obturator neuralgia.
- The patient's pain does not go below the knee, which mitigates against radiculopathy or a more central spinal process.
- The patient's symptoms are unilateral.
- EMG and nerve conduction velocity testing will help delineate the location and degree of nerve compromise if obturator nerve compression is suspected.
- Ultrasound and MRI of the obturator nerve may help identify less common causes of compression of the nerve (e.g., tumor, endometriosis, lipoma, or neural tumors).
- CT imaging may be useful in patients with implants, which would preclude the use of MRI.

Suggested Readings

Dimitropoulos G, Schaepkens van Riempst J, Schertenleib P. Anatomical variation of the obturator nerve: a case report and review of the literature. *J Plastic Reconstr Aesthetic Surg.* 2011;64(7):961—996.

Hasija R, Kelly JJ, Shah NV, et al. Nerve injuries associated with total hip arthroplasty. *J Clin Orthop Trauma.* 2018;9(1):81—86.

Lee B, Stubbs E. Sartorius muscle tear presenting as acute obturator neuralgia. *Clin Imaging.* 2018;51:209—212.

Menderes G, Vilardo N, Schwab CL, et al. Incidental injury and repair of obturator nerve during laparoscopic pelvic lymphadenectomy. *J Minim Invasive Gynecol.* 2016;23(7):S158.

Miklos JR, Moore RD, Chinthakanan O. Obturator neuralgia: a rare complication of tension-free vaginal tape sling—complete resolution after laparoscopic tension-free vaginal tape removal. *J Minim Invasive Gynecol.* 2015;22(4):548.

Moucharafieh R, Wehbe J, Maalouf G. Obturator neuralgia: a result of tight new trendy low cut trousers ('taille basse'). *Int J Surg.* 2008;6(2):164–168.

Osório F, Alves J, Pereira J, et al. Obturator internus muscle endometriosis with nerve involvement: a rare clinical presentation. *J Minim Invasive Gynecol.* 2018;25(2):330–333.

Ueshima H, Myint KZH, Otake H. Detection of large perforating artery by ultrasound prescan before obturator nerve block. *J Clin Anesth.* 2016;29:14.

Waldman SD. Abnormalities of the Obturator Nerve. In: *Comprehensive Atlas of Diagnosis Ultrasound of Painful Conditions.* Philadelphia: Wolters Kluwer; 2016:634–639.

Waldman SD. Obturator Neuralgia. In: *Atlas of Uncommon Pain Syndromes.* 4th ed. Philadelphia: Elsevier; 2020:402–409.

KayLeigh McIlhenny

A 21-Year-Old Female With Right Groin Pain Following a Cheerleading Accident

- Learn the common causes of groin pain (pubalgia).
- Develop an understanding of the innervation of the groin and pelvis.
- Develop an understanding of the anatomy of the adductor tendons.
- Develop an understanding of the causes of adductor tendinitis.
- Learn the clinical presentation of adductor tendinitis.
- Learn how to use physical examination to identify adductor tendinitis.
- Develop an understanding of the treatment options for adductor tendinitis.
- Learn the appropriate testing options to help diagnose adductor tendinitis.
- Learn to identify red flags in patients who present with groin pain.
- Develop an understanding of the role of interventional pain management in the treatment of adductor tendinitis.

KayLeigh McIlhenny

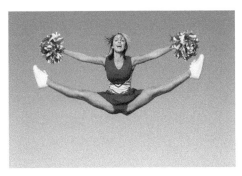

KayLeigh McIlhenny is a 21-year-old cheerleader with the chief complaint of, "I pulled my groin." KayLeigh went on to say that she got hurt at the 'Bama game when she was thrown up into the air and did splits. She felt a sudden, sharp tearing sensation in her right groin and had to be helped off the field. "The good news," KayLeigh said, "is that we won!" The bad news is that she was really having a hard time getting better in spite of massage, acupuncture, aromatherapy, and a lidocaine patch. She said that the pain pills the team doctor gave her seized up her bowels, so she quit taking them.

I asked KayLeigh if she ever had anything like this before, and she shook her head no. She also denied any current urinary or gynecologic symptoms, hematuria, or fever or chills. She also denied a history of kidney stones. Her last menstrual period was about 10 days ago. KayLeigh was using oral contraceptives, but volunteered that the groin pain made sex pretty much impossible. I asked what she was currently doing to manage the pain and she said that "nothing really works." I asked her to rate her pain on a scale of 1 to 10, with 10 being the worst pain she ever had, and she said the pain was a 7 or 8. "Doctor, I have to get back to normal. Cheerleading is my life. The pain is interfering with just about everything. I can't cheerlead, I have a hard time getting dressed, no exercise, no sex—everything. I just really need to get my life back."

I asked KayLeigh to point with one finger to show me where it hurt the most. She pointed to insertions of the adductor tendons at the pubic ramus. She said, "Doc, the pain is right here. This spot right on the bone is really killing on me."

On physical examination, KayLeigh was afebrile. Her respirations were 16. Her pulse was 72 and regular. Her blood pressure (BP) was normal at 118/68. Her head, eyes, ears, nose, throat (HEENT) exam was normal, as was her thyroid examination. Her cardiopulmonary examination was negative. Her abdominal examination revealed no abnormal mass or organomegaly, and no groin mass or hernia was identified. There was no costovertebral angle (CVA) tenderness. There was no peripheral edema. Her low back examination was unremarkable. Her lower extremity neurologic examination was completely normal. The Waldman knee squeeze test was markedly positive (Fig. 11.1).

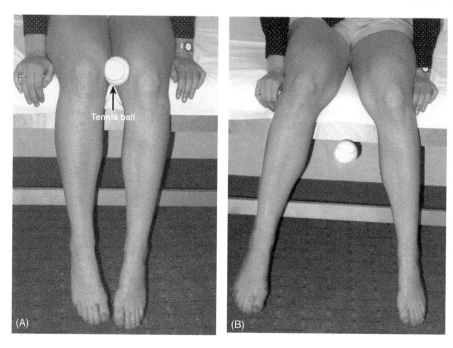

Fig. 11.1 The Waldman knee queeze test is preformed by having the patient place a tennis ball between the knees and gently hold it there. (A) The patient is asked to squeeze the ball as hard as possible. (B) Patients with adductor tendinitis reflexively abduct the knees, causing the tennis ball to fall. (From Waldman SD. *Physical Diagnosis of Pain: An Atlas of Signs and Symptoms.* 3rd ed. St Louis: Elsevier; 2016: Figs. 186-1 and 186-2.)

I asked KayLeigh to lie back on the examination table and let her legs drop apart. She cautiously began abducting her hips and didn't get very far when she cried out in pain. I asked her where it hurt and she again pointed to the origin of the adductor tendons. Visual inspection of the area revealed no ecchymosis. I asked KayLeigh if I could palpate the spot that she identified, and after a moment's hesitation she nodded yes and said, "Sure, just be gentle. It really is sensitive." I said, "No problem. Why don't you hold my hand, and you do the pushing and I'll do the feeling, and together we'll figure out what is going on." She said she liked that idea and relaxed. I had KayLeigh guide my index finger to the spot that was causing the trouble. The spot was right over the origin of the adductor tendons as they inserted on the ischium. I asked KayLeigh to push my finger a little harder and she said, "No way! It already hurts too much." I said, "KayLeigh, I think I know what's going on. How about getting up and walking down the hall for me?" She carefully sat up and slid off the exam table. As she started down the hall, I immediately noticed that she walked cautiously, guarding her right hip.

Key Clinical Points—What's Important and What's Not

THE HISTORY

- A history of recent onset right groin pain following a cheerleading injury
- No history of gynecologic or urinary tract symptoms related to the pain
- No history of kidney stones
- No history of hematuria
- Difficulty in ambulating without reproducing the groin pain
- Difficulty in carrying out activities of daily living
- Pain is localized to the origin of the right adductor tendons
- No fever or chills

THE PHYSICAL EXAMINATION

- The patient is afebrile
- Normal visual inspection of the origin of the right adductor tendons with no ecchymosis
- Palpation of the right adductor tendons elicits pain
- Patient has cautious gait with guarding of the right hip
- The lower extremity neurologic examination is within normal limits

OTHER FINDINGS OF NOTE

- Normal BP
- Normal HEENT examination
- Normal cardiopulmonary examination
- Normal abdominal examination
- No peripheral edema
- No groin mass or inguinal hernia
- No CVA tenderness

What Tests Would You Like to Order?

The following tests were ordered:
- X-ray of the pelvis with special attention to the adductor tendons
- Ultrasound of the pelvis with special attention to the adductor tendons
- Magnetic resonance imaging (MRI) of the pelvis with special attention to the adductor tendons

TEST RESULTS

Plain radiograph of the pelvis demonstrates an avulsion fracture of the ischium (Fig. 11.2). Ultrasound imaging reveals tearing of the adductor tendon near its

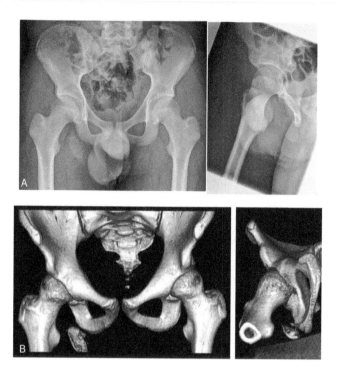

Fig. 11.2 (A) Anteroposterior and lateral radiographs and (B) computed tomography (CT) (3D reconstruction) at time of presentation showing right ischial tuberosity avulsion fracture. (From Ali AM, Lewis A, Sarraf KM. Surgical treatment of an ischial tuberosity avulsion fracture with delayed presentation. *J Clin Orthop Trauma.* 2020;11[1]:S4–S6.)

proximal insertion (Fig. 11.3). MRI of the pelvis reveals hyperintense signal abnormality on coronal and axial fat-saturated T2-weighted images at the origin of the right adductor longus tendon (Fig. 11.4).

 Clinical Correlation—Putting It All Together

What is the diagnosis?
- Adductor tendinitis

The Science Behind the Diagnosis

ANATOMY OF THE ADDUCTOR TENDONS

The adductor muscles of the hip include the adductor longus, adductor brevis, and adductor magnus muscles as well as the gracilis, pectineus, and obturator externus muscles (Figs. 11.5 and 11.6). The adductor function of these muscles is

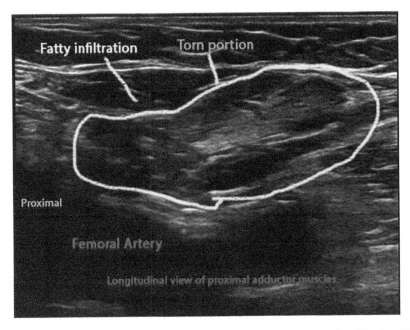

Fig. 11.3 Ultrasound image demonstrating tearing of the proximal adductor tendon. (Courtesy Steven Waldman, MD.)

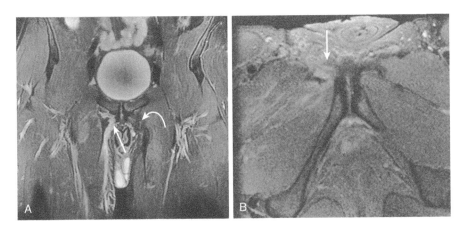

Fig. 11.4 (A) Coronal fat saturated T2-weighted magnetic resonance (MR) image. Hyperintense signal abnormality at the origin of the right adductor longus tendon *(straight arrow)*, consistent with an acute tear. Chronic tear of left adductor longus as evidenced by thickening and hypointensity with retraction of the tendon and healing with scar formation *(curved arrow)*. (B) Axial fat-saturated T2-weighted MR image demonstrating acute right adductor longus tear *(arrow)*. (From MacMahon PJ, Hogan BA, Shelly MJ, et al. Imaging of groin pain. *Magn Reson Imaging Clin N Am.* 2009;17: 655–666.)

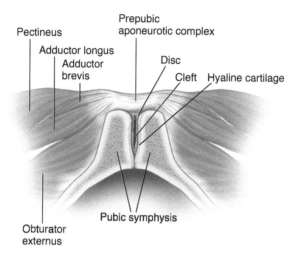

Fig. 11.5 Axial section through the pubic symphysis below the level of the pubic crest, demonstrating the anatomy of the adductor muscles. Note the origin of these muscles from the prepubic aponeurotic complex, which is an extension of the underlying fibrocartilaginous pubic symphysis. (From Waldman SD. *Atlas of Pain Management Injection Techniques.* 4th ed. St Louis: Elsevier; 2017: Fig. 111-5.)

innervated by the obturator nerve, which is susceptible to trauma from pelvic fractures and compression by tumor. The tendons of the adductor muscles of the hip have their origin along the pubis and ischial ramus, and it is at this point that tendinitis frequently occurs.

CLINICAL SYNDROME

The increased use of exercise equipment in gyms for lower extremity strengthening has resulted in an increased incidence of adductor tendinitis (Fig. 11.7). The adductor muscles of the hip include the gracilis, adductor longus, adductor brevis, and adductor magnus muscles. The adductor function of these muscles is innervated by the obturator nerve, which is susceptible to trauma from pelvic fractures and compression by tumor. The tendons of the adductor muscles of the hip have their origin along the pubis and ischial ramus, and it is at this point that tendinitis frequently occurs (see Fig. 11.5).

These tendons and their associated muscles are susceptible to the development of tendinitis owing to overuse or trauma secondary to stretch injuries. Inciting factors include the vigorous use of exercise equipment for lower extremity strengthening and acute stretching of the musculotendinous units as a result of sports injuries, such as sliding into bases when playing baseball.

The pain of adductor tendinitis is sharp, constant, and severe, with sleep disturbance often reported. The patient may attempt to splint the inflamed tendons

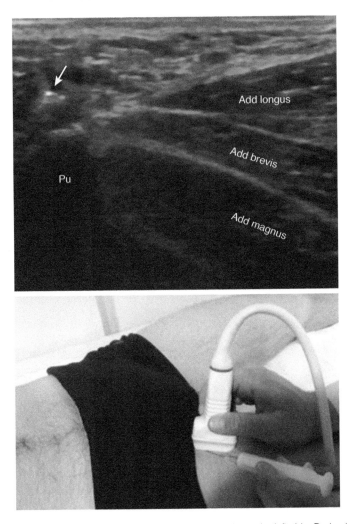

Fig. 11.6 A 19-year-old male runner who experienced groin pain on the left side. During local platelet-rich plasma injection with the direct out-of-plane technique, the tip of the needle *(arrow)* is observed next to the origin of the adductor muscles. The exemplary photograph shows the positioning of the needle and the transducer for such an injection. The needle may or may not be touching the transducer, depending on the injection technique and the sterility of the gel. *Pu*, Pubic bone; *Add*, adductor. (From Özçakar L, Utku B. Ultrasound images of groin pain in the athlete: a pictorial essay. *PM&R.* 2014;6[8]:753–756.)

by adopting an adductor lurch type of gait—shifting the trunk of the body over the affected extremity when walking. In addition to the previously described pain, patients with adductor tendinitis often experience a gradual decrease in functional ability, with decreasing hip range of motion making simple everyday

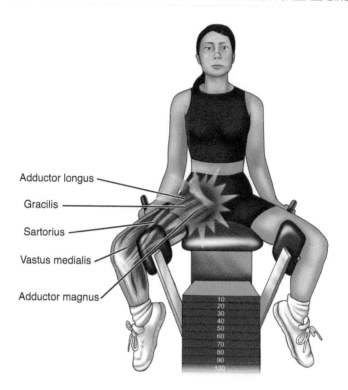

Adductor longus

Gracilis

Sartorius

Vastus medialis

Adductor magnus

Fig. 11.7 The patient with adductor tendinitis reports pain on palpation of the origins of the adductor tendons. Active resisted adduction and passive abduction reproduce the pain. (From Waldman SD. *Atlas of Uncommon Pain Syndromes.* 4th ed. Philadelphia: Saunders; 2020: Fig. 108.1.)

tasks such as getting in or out of an automobile quite difficult. With continued disuse, muscle wasting may occur, and an adhesive capsulitis of the hip may develop.

SIGNS AND SYMPTOMS

On physical examination, a patient with adductor tendinitis reports pain on palpation of the origins of the adductor tendons. Active resisted adduction and passive abduction reproduce the pain. Patients with adductor tendinitis also exhibit a positive Waldman knee squeeze test for adductor tendinitis (see Fig. 11.1). Tendinitis of the musculotendinous unit of the hip frequently coexists with bursitis of the associated bursa of the hip joint, creating additional pain and functional disability. Neurologic examination of the hip and lower extremity is normal, unless there has been concomitant stretch injury to the plexus or obturator nerve.

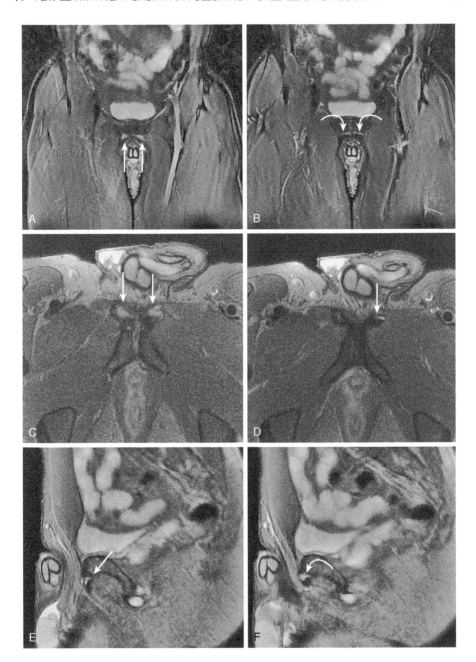

Fig. 11.8 (A) Coronal fat-saturated T2-weighted magnetic resonance (MR) image. Bilateral severe adductor longus origin tendinosis *(arrows)*. (B) Coronal fat-saturated T2-weighted MR image. Bilateral secondary clefts extend from the pubic symphysis into the adductor attachments, indicating some disruption of the prepubic aponeurotic complex tissue *(curved arrows)*. (C) Axial fat-saturated T2-weighted MR image demonstrating bilateral adductor longus tendinosis *(arrows)*. (D) Three-dimensional axial fat-saturated T2-weighted MR image. Small tear of the left adductor longus tendon *(arrow)*. (E) Sagittal fat-saturated T2-weighted MR image. Small tears of the origin of the left adductor

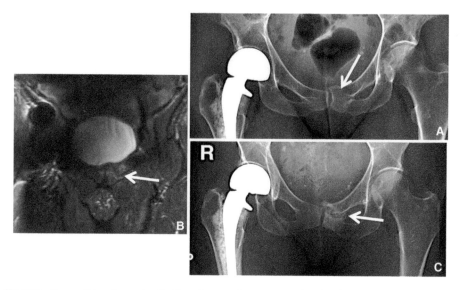

Fig. 11.9 Sequential radiographs (A, C) and magnetic resonance imaging (MRI) of the pelvis (B) in a 75-year-old woman with a right hip hemiarthroplasty and a left pubic symphysis insufficiency fracture. Initial radiograph (A) was obtained after a low-energy fall from less than standing height and persistent pain. Suspicion for fracture led to the MRI, which demonstrated a mildly displaced and impacted superior pubic ramus fracture (B). Radiograph obtained 3 months after the fall shows healing pubic symphysis fracture with callus formation. (From Link TM. Radiology of osteoporosis. *Can Assoc Radiol J*. 2016;67[1]:28–40 [Fig. 4].)

TESTING

Plain radiographs are indicated in all patients with hip, thigh, and groin pain (see Fig. 11.2). Based on the patient's clinical presentation, additional tests, including complete blood cell count, erythrocyte sedimentation rate, and antinuclear antibody testing, may be indicated. MRI and ultrasound imaging of the hip and pelvis are indicated if aseptic necrosis or occult mass is suspected and to help confirm the diagnosis (Fig. 11.8). Radionucleotide bone scanning should be considered if the possibility of occult fracture of the pelvis is being considered. Electromyography can help rule out compression neuropathy or trauma of the obturator nerve and rule out plexopathy and radiculopathy. Injection at the insertion of the adductor tendons serves as both a diagnostic and a therapeutic maneuver.

◀ longus tendon *(arrow)*. (F) Sagittal fat-saturated T2-weighted MR image. This image demonstrates more severe adductor longus tendinosis that involves the prepubic aponeurotic complex *(curved arrow)*. (From MacMahon PJ, Hogan BA, Shelly MJ, et al. Imaging of groin pain. *Magn Reson Imaging Clin N Am*. 2009;17:655–666.)

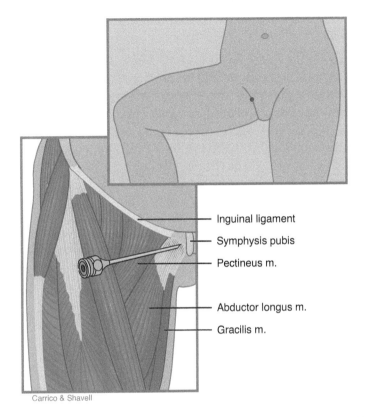

Inguinal ligament
Symphysis pubis
Pectineus m.

Abductor longus m.
Gracilis m.

Carrico & Shavell

Fig. 11.10 Injection of the origin of the adductor tendons. *m*, muscle. (From Waldman SD. *Atlas of Pain Management Injection Techniques.* 4th ed. St Louis: Elsevier; 2017: Fig. 111-4.)

DIFFERENTIAL DIAGNOSIS

Internal derangement of the hip may mimic the clinical presentation of adductor tendinitis. Occasionally, indirect inguinal hernia can produce pain that can be confused with adductor tendinitis. If trauma has occurred, consideration of the possibility of occult pelvic fracture, especially in individuals with osteopenia or osteoporosis, should be entertained, and plain radiographs, radionucleotide bone scanning, and MRI should be obtained (Fig. 11.9). Avascular necrosis of the hip also may produce hip pain that can mimic the clinical presentation of adductor tendinitis. Entrapment neuropathy or stretch injury to the ilioinguinal, genitofemoral, and obturator nerves and plexopathy and radiculopathy should be considered if the physical finding of neurologic deficit is identified in patients thought to have adductor tendinitis because all of these clinical entities may coexist.

TREATMENT

Initial treatment of the pain and functional disability associated with adductor tendinitis should include a combination of nonsteroidal antiinflammatory drugs (NSAIDs) or cyclooxygenase-2 inhibitors and physical therapy. Local application of heat and cold may be beneficial. For patients who do not respond to these treatment modalities, injection at the insertion of the adductor tendons of the hip with a local anesthetic and steroid may be a reasonable next step (Fig. 11.10). The use of ultrasound guidance may improve the accuracy of needle placement and decrease the incidence of needle-related complications.

Physical modalities, including local heat and gentle stretching exercises, should be introduced several days after the patient undergoes injection. Vigorous exercises should be avoided because they will exacerbate patient symptoms. Simple analgesics, NSAIDs, and antimyotonic agents such as tizanidine may be used concurrently with this injection technique.

HIGH-YIELD TAKEAWAYS

- The patient's symptomatology began after a cheerleading accident.
- The patient's pain is localized to the origin of the left adductor tendons.
- The patient has a positive Waldman knee squeeze test, which is highly suggestive of adductor tendinitis.
- The patient is afebrile, making an acute infectious etiology (e.g., postoperative infection or urosepsis) unlikely.
- The lower extremity neurologic examination is within normal limits, making a central spinal or lumbar plexus lesion much less likely.
- The X-ray of the adductor tendons demonstrates characteristic findings, as does the MRI and ultrasound imaging.

Suggested Readings

Damme KV, De Coster L, Mermuys K, et al. Bone scan findings in calcific tendinitis at the gluteus maximus insertion: some illustrative cases. *Radiol Case Rep.* 2017;12 (1):168–174.

Hölmich P. Groin injuries in athletes—new stepping stones. *Sports Orthop Traumatol.* 2017;33(2):106–112.

Özçakar L, Utku B. Ultrasound images of groin pain in the athlete: a pictorial essay. *PM&R.* 2014;6(8):753–756.

Waldman SD. Adductor tendinitis. In: *Atlas of Uncommon Pain Syndromes.* 4th ed. Philadelphia: Elsevier; 2018:297–300.

Waldman SD. Injection technique for adductor tendinitis. In: *Atlas of Pain Management Injection Techniques*. 4th ed. Philadelphia: Elsevier; 2017:395–399.

Waldman SD. The Waldman knee squeeze test for adductor tendinitis. In: *Physical Diagnosis of Pain*. 3rd ed. Philadelphia: Elsevier; 2016:286–288.

Waldman SD, Campbell RSD. Adductor tendinitis. In: *Imaging of Pain*. Philadelphia: Saunders Elsevier; 2011:355–356.

Ashley Stubbs

A 32-Year-Old Male With a Dull Ache in the Buttock and Pain Down the Back of the Thigh and Calf After a Fall on the Ice

LEARNING OBJECTIVES

- Learn the common causes of lower extremity pain.
- Develop an understanding of the anatomy of the sciatic nerve.
- Develop an understanding of the unique relationship of the sciatic nerve to the piriformis muscle.
- Develop an understanding of the causes of piriformis syndrome.
- Develop an understanding of the differential diagnosis of lower extremity pain and numbness.
- Learn the clinical presentation of piriformis syndrome.
- Learn the dermatomes of the lower extremity.
- Learn how to use physical examination to identify piriformis syndrome.
- Develop an understanding of the treatment options for piriformis syndrome.

Ashley Stubbs

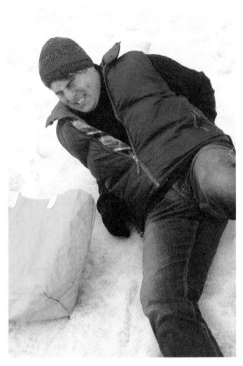

Ashley Stubbs is a 32-year-old chief of security for a tech firm with the chief complaint of, "Ever since I fell on the ice, I've had a pain in my butt that goes down the back of my right leg." Ashley stated that a couple of months ago, as he was walking back from the corner bodega, he slipped on an icy patch and fell hard onto his right buttock. He said that he lay there for a few moments and then carefully got to his feet. He felt around and didn't think he broke anything so he carefully made his way home. By the time he got home, his butt was really hurting. He looked in the mirror and saw that a large bruise was beginning to form. He took a couple of aspirin and got out the heating pad. The next morning, he felt like he had been hit by a car, and in addition to the bruise, he now had a large, tender lump in the center of his right buttock. It really hurt, but he toughed through it. Over the next couple of weeks, the bruise got better, as did the lump, but the pain actually got worse and at times the top of his foot felt like it was asleep. "Doctor, I consider myself a pretty tough guy. You know, I was in the Special Forces, but this is literally kicking my ass. Fortunately, most of my day is in the office, but I don't know what I would do if I had to be back out in the field. Sitting is bad enough, but I seriously can't run, and going up stairs is a bitch. I can't believe I fell on the ice—so stupid!"

I asked Ashley if he had experienced any pain, numbness, or weakness in his left leg and he just shook his head and replied, "Doc, the pain is all on the right—the side that I fell on. You know, over the last couple of weeks, I feel like my right leg is getting weaker. Maybe it's just the fact that I am off my exercise routine, but I have really started having trouble walking up the stairs." "Do both legs feel weak?" I asked. He said "No, just the right." I asked Ashley what he had tried to make it better and he said that he felt like the heating pad and sleeping on his left side with a pillow between his legs

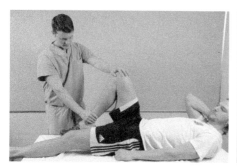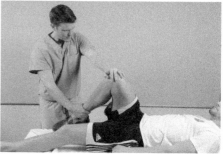

Fig. 12.1   (A, B) The piriformis test. (From Waldman SD. *Physical Diagnosis of Pain: An Atlas of Signs and Symptoms*. 3rd ed. St Louis: Elsevier; 2016: Figs. 190-2 and 190-3.)

helped a little, but he was having trouble sitting for long periods of time and felt the need to get up every 10 to 15 minutes to avoid the pain getting too strong. "Also, a Tylenol PM with a beer chaser seemed to help some, at least with sleep."

I asked Ashley to show me where the pain was and he pointed to his right buttock and then traced his hand down his posterior thigh all the way to the posterior calf. "Once in a while, if I sit too long, like when I'm in a meeting with the boss, the pain can go all the way down to my foot. I've got to tell you, that's no fun." I asked Ashley about any fever, chills, or other constitutional symptoms such as weight loss, night sweats, etc., and he shook his head no. He denied any musculoskeletal or systemic symptoms.

On physical examination, Ashley was afebrile. His respirations were 18, his pulse was 74 and regular, and his blood pressure was 124/76. Ashley's head, eyes, ears, nose, throat (HEENT) exam was normal, as was his thyroid exam. Auscultation of his carotids revealed no bruits, and the pulses in all four extremities were normal. He had a regular rhythm without abnormal beats. His cardiac exam was otherwise unremarkable. His abdominal examination revealed no abnormal mass or organomegaly. There was no peripheral edema. His low back examination was unremarkable, although flexion of the lumbar spine caused some pain in the right buttock. There was no costovertebral angle (CVA) tenderness. Visual inspection of the right buttock and lower extremity was unremarkable. There was no rubor or color and no evidence of ecchymosis. Palpation of the sciatic notch caused Ashley to say, "You're right on it, Doc. That's it." I performed the piriformis test as well as the heel contralateral knee test, which were both markedly positive (Figs. 12.1 and 12.2).

A careful neurologic examination of both lower extremities revealed a mildly decreased sensation in the distribution of the right sciatic nerve and marked weakness of the right gluteal muscles (Fig. 12.3). Deep tendon reflexes were physiologic throughout. There was a positive Tinel sign over the right sciatic nerve.

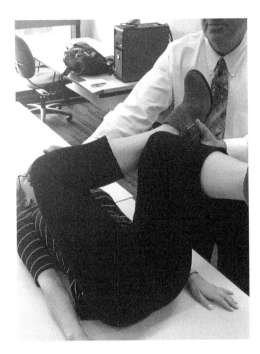

Fig. 12.2 The patient is asked to place the heel of the painful leg above the contralateral knee. The examiner then straightens the leg as much as possible with the heel of the affected leg kept above the contralateral knee. (Courtesy Steven Waldman, MD.)

Key Clinical Points—What's Important and What's Not

THE HISTORY

- A history of the onset of severe right buttock, posterior thigh, posterior calf, and foot pain immediately following a fall on the ice
- Right foot feels like it is falling asleep
- The right leg feels weak
- Difficulty walking up stairs
- Pain made worse with sitting and walking
- No symptoms in the left lower extremity
- No fever or chills
- History of recent trauma

THE PHYSICAL EXAMINATION

- The patient is afebrile
- Marked weakness of the gluteal muscles on the right
- Numbness in the distribution of the sciatic nerve on the right (see Fig. 12.3)
- Tenderness over sciatic notch
- Positive piriformis test (see Fig. 12.1)

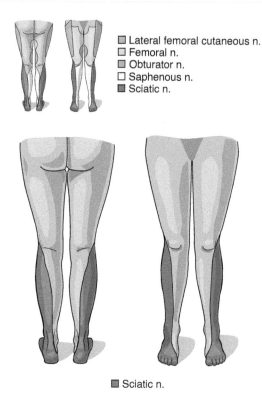

☐ Lateral femoral cutaneous n.
☐ Femoral n.
☐ Obturator n.
☐ Saphenous n.
☑ Sciatic n.

☑ Sciatic n.

Fig. 12.3 The sensory distribution of the sciatic nerve. *n*, nerve. (From Waldman SD. *Atlas of Interventional Pain Management*. 4th ed. Philadelphia: Saunders; 2015: Fig. 128.8.)

- Positive heel contralateral knee test (see Fig. 12.2)
- Positive Tinel sign over the sciatic nerve on the right
- No motor deficit in the left lower extremity
- Deep tendon reflexes within normal limits

OTHER FINDINGS OF NOTE

- Normal HEENT examination
- Normal cardiovascular examination
- Normal pulmonary examination
- Normal abdominal examination
- No peripheral edema

 What Tests Would You Like to Order?

The following tests were ordered:
- Ultrasound of the right sciatic nerve at the level of the piriformis muscle

- Magnetic resonance imaging (MRI) of the pelvis with special attention to the right sciatic nerve
- Electromyography (EMG) and nerve conduction velocity testing of the right sciatic nerve

TEST RESULTS

Ultrasound examination of the sciatic nerve at the level of the sciatic triangle reveals no obvious tumor or mass compressing the sciatic nerve. MRI of the pelvis, EMG, and nerve conduction velocity testing revealed normal needle examination of the muscles above the piriformis muscle and abnormal below the piriformis muscles.

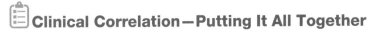 Clinical Correlation—Putting It All Together

What is the diagnosis?
- Piriformis syndrome secondary to acute trauma to the right buttock

The Science Behind the Diagnosis
ANATOMY

The sciatic nerve provides innervation to the distal lower extremity and foot with the exception of the medial aspect of the calf and foot, which are subserved by the saphenous nerve. The largest nerve in the body, the sciatic nerve is derived from the L4, L5, and S1–S3 nerve roots (Fig. 12.4). The roots fuse in front of the anterior surface of the lateral sacrum on the anterior surface of the piriformis muscle (Fig. 12.5). The nerve travels inferiorly and leaves the pelvis just below the piriformis muscle via the sciatic notch (Figs. 12.6 and 12.7). Just beneath the nerve at this point is the obturator internus muscle. The sciatic nerve lies anterior to the gluteus maximus muscle; at this muscle's lower border, the sciatic nerve lies halfway between the greater trochanter and the ischial tuberosity. The sciatic nerve courses downward past the lesser trochanter to lie posterior and medial to the femur. In the midthigh, the nerve gives off branches to the hamstring muscles and the adductor magnus muscle. In most patients, the nerve divides to form the tibial and common peroneal nerves in the upper portion of the popliteal fossa, although in some patients these nerves can remain separate through their entire course. The tibial nerve continues downward to provide innervation to the distal lower extremity, whereas the common peroneal nerve travels laterally to innervate a portion of the knee joint and, via its lateral cutaneous branch, provides sensory innervation to the back and lateral side of the upper calf.

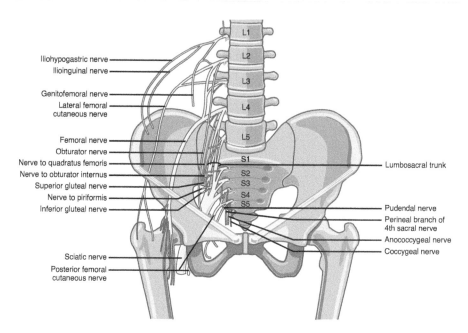

Fig. 12.4 The largest nerve in the body, the sciatic nerve is derived from the L4, L5, and S1–S3 nerve roots. (From Waldman SD. *Atlas of Interventional Pain Management.* 4th ed. Philadelphia: Saunders; 2015: Fig. 128-3.)

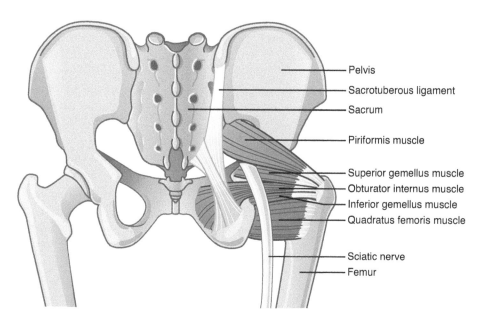

Fig. 12.5 The nerve roots that make up the sciatic nerve fuse in front of the anterior surface of the lateral sacrum on the anterior surface of the piriformis muscle. (From Waldman SD. *Atlas of Interventional Pain Management.* 4th ed. Philadelphia: Saunders; 2015: Fig. 128-4.)

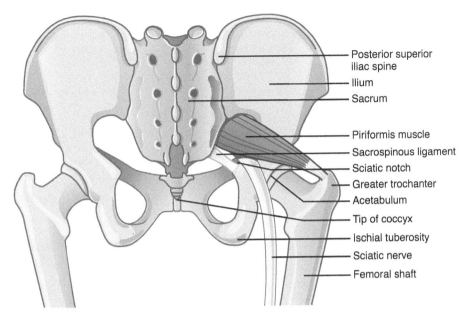

Posterior superior
iliac spine

Ilium

Sacrum

Piriformis muscle

Sacrospinous ligament

Sciatic notch

Greater trochanter

Acetabulum

Tip of coccyx

Ischial tuberosity

Sciatic nerve

Femoral shaft

Fig. 12.6   The sciatic nerve travels inferiorly and leaves the pelvis just below the piriformis muscle via the sciatic notch. (From Waldman SD. *Atlas of Interventional Pain Management*. 4th ed. Philadelphia: Saunders; 2015: Fig. 128-6.)

The piriformis muscle has its origin from the anterior sacrum. It passes laterally through the greater sciatic foramen to insert on the upper border of the greater trochanter of the femur (Fig. 12.8; see Fig. 12.7). The piriformis muscle's primary function is to externally rotate the femur at the hip joint. The piriformis muscle is innervated by the sacral plexus. With internal rotation of the femur, the tendinous insertion and belly of the muscle can compress the sciatic nerve and, if this persists, cause entrapment of the sciatic nerve (Fig. 12.9).

CLINICAL SYNDROME

An uncommon cause of sciatica, piriformis syndrome is caused by entrapment and compression of the sciatic nerve by the piriformis muscle at the level of the sciatic notch (see Fig. 12.7). Patients suffering from piriformis syndrome complain of pain that begins in the buttock and radiates into the affected leg all the way to the foot (Fig. 12.10). There is associated numbness and dysesthesias as well as weakness in the distribution of the sciatic nerve. As the syndrome progresses, the patient may experience altered gait as a result of the pain and weakness associated with the compromise of the sciatic nerve. This alteration of gait will often cause secondary sacroiliac, low back, and hip pain, which may serve to confuse the diagnosis. Untreated, atrophy of the muscles innervated by the

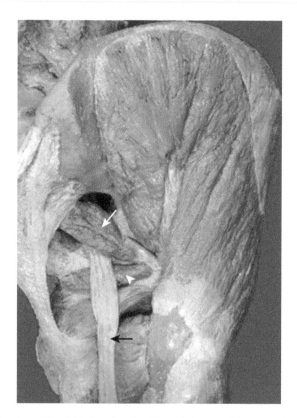

Fig. 12.7 Posterior view of the right gluteal region. The sciatic nerve *(black arrow)* passes through the infrapiriform foramen, bordered superiorly by the piriformis muscle *(white arrow)* and inferiorly by the portion of the obturator internus muscle that is outside the pelvis *(arrowhead)*. (From Waldman SD. *Physical Diagnosis of Pain: An Atlas of Signs and Symptoms.* 3rd ed. St Louis: Elsevier; 2016: Fig. 190-1.)

sciatic nerve may result. Piriformis syndrome is the clinical constellation of symptoms that occurs when the sciatic nerve is compressed and/or entrapped. The cause of this sciatic nerve compromise can be from a variety of pathologic processes: direct trauma to the nerve; compression of the nerve by tumor, hematoma or mass; and compression of the nerve by hypertrophied or anomalous piriformis muscle (Figs. 12.11, 12.12, and 12.13).

Piriformis syndrome is frequently misdiagnosed as lumbar radiculopathy or is attributed to primary hip pathology, leading to both diagnostic and therapeutic misadventures. Plain radiographs of the hip will help identify primary hip pathology, and EMG will help distinguish the compromise of sciatic nerve function associated with piriformis syndrome from radiculopathy. Most patients who suffer from lumbar radiculopathy have back pain associated with reflex, motor, and sensory changes that are associated with back pain, whereas patients with piriformis syndrome have only secondary back pain and no reflex changes.

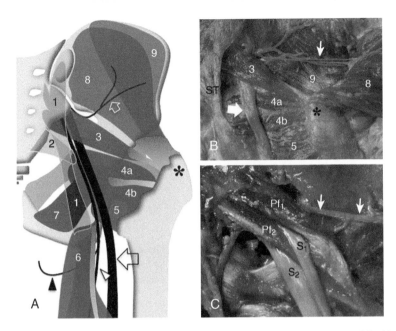

Fig. 12.8 Anatomy of the sciatic nerve. (A) Schematic drawing of the posterior aspect of the hip showing relevant regional structures, including the sacrotuberous (1) and sacrospinous (2) ligaments, the piriformis (3), the superior (4a) and inferior (4b) gemellus, the quadratus femoris (5), the hamstrings (6), the obturator internus (7), and the gluteus medius (8) and minimus (9), which insert into the greater trochanter *(asterisk)*. The sciatic nerve *(open black arrow)* exits the pelvis, passing through the greater sciatic foramen as individual tibial (medial) and peroneal (lateral) components embedded in a common nerve sheath. It then continues down, passing deep to the piriformis and lateral to the conjoined tendon of the long head of the biceps and semitendinosus. The superior gluteal nerve *(open white arrow)* leaves the pelvis through the sciatic foramen above the piriformis and then divides into a superior and an inferior branch. The posterior femoral cutaneous nerve descends alongside the medial aspect of the sciatic nerve, accompanied by the inferior gluteal artery. After sending branches for the lower gluteus maximus and overlying skin, this nerve divides into a perineal *(black arrowhead)* and a descending *(white arrowhead)* branch. (B) Corresponding cadaveric specimen of the posterior hip after removal of the gluteus maximus showing the insertions of the piriformis (3), superior (4a) and inferior (4b) gemellus, quadratus femoris (5), and gluteus medius (8) and minimus (9) on the greater trochanter *(asterisk)*. Note the piriformis muscle covering the greater sciatic foramen and intervening between the superior gluteal neurovascular bundle and the sciatic nerve. *ST*, Sacrotuberous ligament. (C) Cadaveric specimen of a double-headed piriformis muscle *(Pf₁ and Pf₂)*. There is a high division of the sciatic nerve with its lateral component *(S₁)* passing in between the two bellies of the muscle and the medial component *(S₂)* crossing the muscle inferiorly. Note the superior gluteal nerve *(white arrows)*. (From Martinoli C, Miguel-Perez M, Padua L, et al. Imaging of neuropathies about the hip. *Eur J Radiol.* 2013;82[1]:17–26.)

Furthermore, the motor and sensory changes of piriformis syndrome are limited to the distribution of the sciatic nerve below the sciatic notch. Lumbar radiculopathy and sciatic nerve entrapment may coexist as the so-called "double crush" syndrome, which can further confuse the clinical picture. Based on the patient's clinical presentation, additional testing may be indicated, including complete

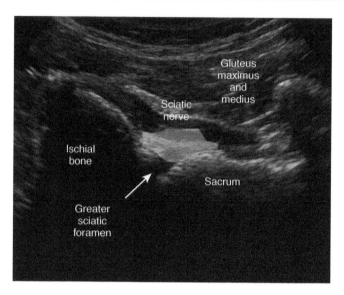

Fig. 12.9 Transverse ultrasound image showing the curved hyperechoic margins of the sacrum and ischial bone. The sciatic nerve is visualized as a flattened hyperechoic structure lying between the hyperechoic curves of the sacrum and ischium. (From Waldman SD. *Atlas of Interventional Pain Management*. 4th ed. Philadelphia: Saunders; 2015: Fig. 128-15.)

blood cell count, uric acid, sedimentation rate, and antinuclear antibody testing. MRI or computed tomography (CT) scanning of the lumbar spine is indicated if a herniated disk, spinal stenosis, or a space-occupying lesion is suspected. Piriformis injection technique with local anesthetic and/or steroid can be utilized as both a diagnostic and a therapeutic maneuver (Fig. 12.14).

SIGNS AND SYMPTOMS

Patients suffering from piriformis syndrome will exhibit tenderness on palpation of the sciatic notch. A positive straight leg raising test is often present, as is a positive Tinel sign when the sciatic nerve is percussed at the sciatic notch. The pain of piriformis syndrome may be elicited by the piriformis syndrome provocation test. To perform the piriformis syndrome provocation test, the patient is placed in the modified Sims position with the affected leg superior. The hip of the affected leg is then flexed approximately 50 degrees and, while stabilizing the pelvis, the affected leg is pushed downward (see Fig. 12.1). The test is considered positive if the patient's pain symptomatology is reproduced. On palpation of the piriformis muscle, a swollen, indurated muscle belly may be appreciated. Weakness of the affected gluteal muscles and muscle wasting may be identified in more advanced cases of untreated piriformis syndrome.

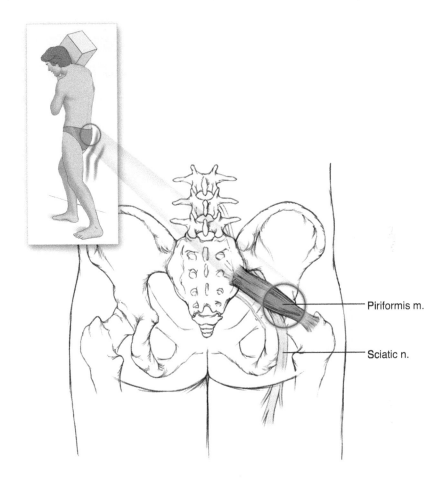

Fig. 12.10   Patients suffering from piriformis syndrome complain of pain that begins in the buttock and radiates into the affected leg all the way to the foot. There may be associated numbness and dysesthesias as well as weakness in the distribution of the sciatic nerve. *m*, muscle; *n*, nerve. (From Waldman SD. *Atlas of Common Pain Syndromes*. 4th ed. Philadelphia: Elsevier; 2019: Fig. 90-4.)

TESTING

EMG can help distinguish lumbar radiculopathy from piriformis syndrome. Plain radiographs of the back, hip, and pelvis are indicated in all patients who present with piriformis syndrome to rule out occult bony disorders. Based on the patient's clinical presentation, additional testing may be warranted, including a complete blood count, uric acid level, erythrocyte sedimentation rate, and antinuclear antibody testing. MRI of the back is indicated if herniated disk, spinal stenosis, or space-occupying lesion is suspected. MRI and ultrasound imaging of the hip and piriformis muscle may elucidate the cause of compression of the sciatic nerve (Fig. 12.15; see Figs. 12.12 and 12.13). Injection in the region of the sciatic nerve at this level serves as both a diagnostic and a therapeutic maneuver.

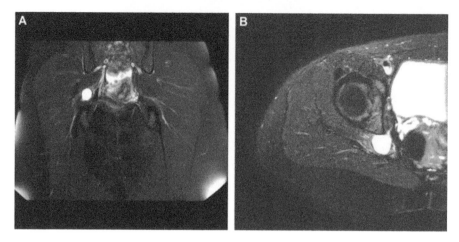

Fig. 12.11 Magnetic resonance imaging (MRI) findings of a 32-year-old female patient. Coronal (A) and axial (B) MRI images demonstrating about an approximately 2-cm multilobulated cystic mass located in the piriformis muscle that showed high intensity on T2-weighted and low intensity on T1-weighted image. (From Park JH, Jeong HJ, Shin HK, et al. Piriformis ganglion: an uncommon cause of sciatica. *Orthop Traumatol Surg Res.* 2016;102(2):257–260.)

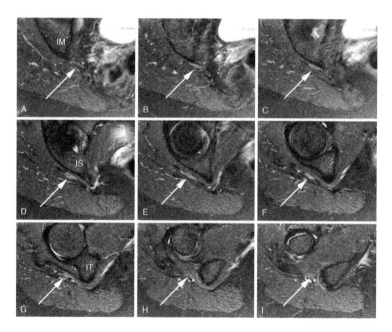

Fig. 12.12 Typical findings of irritative abnormalities of the sciatic nerve in piriformis syndrome (nerve perpendicular oblique view, magnetic resonance neurographic acquisition sequence). (A) The sciatic nerve is bowed over the medial surface of the piriformis muscle. (B) Nerve image intensity increases as the nerve passes between the piriformis tendon and the ischial margin. (C–F) The image intensity increase persists as the nerve descends through the ischial tunnel. (G–I) Nerve image intensity progressively normalizes, with the nerve becoming isointense with surrounding muscle as it descends into the upper thigh. Arrows indicate the sciatic nerve. *IM,* Ischial margin; *IS,* ischial spine; *IT,* ischial tuberosity. (From Filler AG. Piriformis and related entrapment syndromes: diagnosis and management. *Neurosurg Clin N Am.* 2008;19[4]:609–622.)

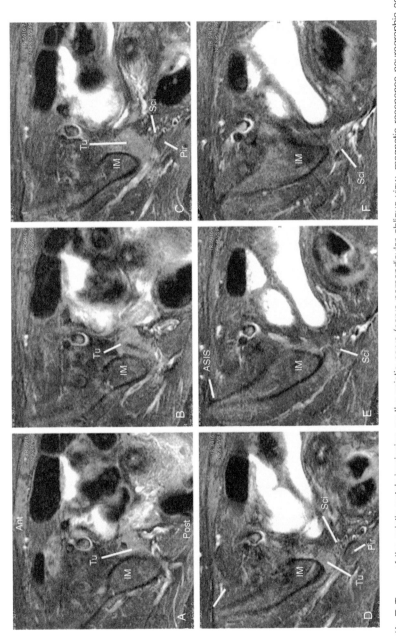

Fig. 12.13 (A–F) Tumor of the sciatic notch impinging on the sciatic nerve (nerve perpendicular oblique view, magnetic resonance neurographic acquisition sequence). *Ant,* Anterior; *ASIS,* anterior superior iliac spine; *IC,* iliac crest; *IM,* ischial margin; *Pir,* piriformis muscle; *Post,* posterior; *Sci,* sciatic nerve; *Tu,* tumor. (From Filler AG. Piriformis and related entrapment syndromes: diagnosis and management. *Neurosurg Clin N Am.* 2008;19[4]:609–622.)

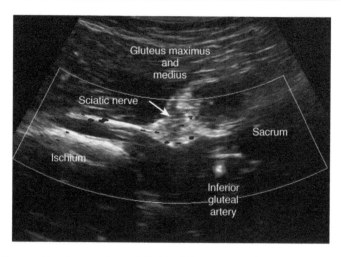

Fig. 12.14 Ultrasound imaging may be useful in identifying tumors and masses that may be responsible for the symptoms of piriformis syndrome. (From Waldman SD. *Atlas of Interventional Pain Management*. 4th ed. Philadelphia: Saunders; 2015: Fig. 128-16.)

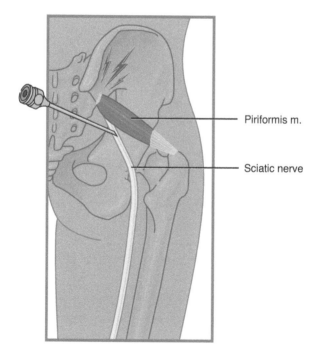

Fig. 12.15 Injection technique for piriformis syndrome. *m*, muscle. (From Waldman SD. *Atlas of Pain Management Injection Techniques*. 4th ed. St Louis: Elsevier; 2017: Fig. 125-4.)

DIFFERENTIAL DIAGNOSIS

Piriformis syndrome is often misdiagnosed as lumbar radiculopathy or primary hip disease; radiographs of the hip and EMG can make the distinction. In addition, most patients with lumbar radiculopathy have back pain associated with reflex, motor, and sensory changes, whereas patients with piriformis syndrome have only secondary back pain and no reflex changes. The motor and sensory changes of piriformis syndrome are limited to the distribution of the sciatic nerve below the sciatic notch. Lumbar radiculopathy and sciatic nerve entrapment may coexist as the double-crush syndrome.

TREATMENT

Initial treatment of the pain and functional disability associated with piriformis syndrome includes a combination of nonsteroidal antiinflammatory drugs or cyclooxygenase-2 inhibitors and physical therapy. The local application of heat and cold may also be beneficial. Any repetitive activity that may exacerbate patient symptoms should be avoided. If the patient is a side sleeper, then placing a pillow between the legs may be helpful. If the patient is suffering from significant paresthesias, gabapentin may be added. For patients who do not respond to these treatment modalities, injection of local anesthetic and methylprednisolone in the region of the sciatic nerve at the level of the piriformis muscle is a reasonable next step. Ultrasound needle guidance will improve the accuracy of needle placement and decrease the incidence of needle-induced complications (see Fig. 12.15). Rarely, surgical release of the entrapment is required to obtain relief.

HIGH-YIELD TAKEAWAYS

- The patient is afebrile, making an acute infectious etiology unlikely.
- The patient's symptomatology is most likely due to trauma to the piriformis muscle and underlying sciatic nerve from a fall onto the right buttock.
- Physical examination and testing should be focused on identification of other pathologic processes that may mimic the clinical diagnosis of piriformis syndrome.
- The patient exhibits the neurologic and physical examination findings that are highly suggestive of piriformis syndrome.
- The patient's symptoms are unilateral.
- EMG and nerve conduction velocity testing will help delineate the location and degree of nerve compromise if sciatic nerve compression is suspected.
- Ultrasound and MRI of the sciatic nerve may help identify less common causes of compression of the nerve (e.g., tumor, lipoma, or neural tumors).

Suggested Readings

Fritz J, Chhabra A, Wang KC, et al. Magnetic resonance neurography—guided nerve blocks for the diagnosis and treatment of chronic pelvic pain syndrome. *Neuroimaging Clin N Am.* 2014;24(1):211–234.

Michel F, Decavel P, Toussirot E, et al. The piriformis muscle syndrome: an exploration of anatomical context, pathophysiological hypotheses and diagnostic criteria. *Ann Phys Rehab Med.* 2013;56(4):300–311.

Park JH, Jeong HJ, Shin HK, et al. Piriformis ganglion: an uncommon cause of sciatica. *Orthop Traumatol Surg Res.* 2016;102(2):257–260.

Waldman SD. Injection technique for piriformis syndrome. In: *Pain Review.* 2nd ed. Philadelphia: Elsevier; 2017:531.

Waldman SD. Piriformis syndrome. In: *Pain Review.* 2nd ed. Philadelphia: Elsevier; 2017:297–298.

Waldman SD. Ultrasound-guided injection technique for piriformis syndrome. In: *Comprehensive Atlas of Ultrasound Guided Pain Management Injection Techniques.* Philadelphia: Lippincott; 2014:824–834.

13

Carrie Matheson

A 30-Year-Old Female With Shooting Rectal Pain

- Learn the common causes of rectal pain.
- Develop an understanding of the anatomy of the nerves of the rectum and pelvis.
- Develop an understanding of the etiology of proctalgia fugax.
- Learn the clinical presentation of proctalgia fugax.
- Learn how to use physical examination to rule out pathology and other urogenital pain syndromes that may mimic proctalgia fugax.
- Develop an understanding of the treatment options for proctalgia fugax.
- Learn the appropriate testing options to help diagnose proctalgia fugax.
- Learn to identify red flags in patients who present with rectal pain.

Carrie Matheson

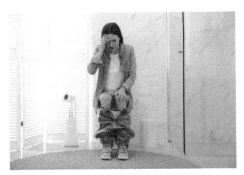

Carrie Matheson is a 30-year-old graphic designer with the chief complaint of, "I've got shooting pain in my rectum that just won't go away." Carrie went on to say that the rectal pain came on suddenly about 6 months ago. She was unable to identify any antecedent rectal or pelvic trauma or abnormalities associated with the onset of her pain, but did volunteer that she had been under a lot of stress at work. Carrie denied any urinary tract or vaginal infections or any gastrointestinal disturbance, constipation, or change in bowel habits. Carrie described the pain as sudden, excruciating, shooting pains located deep in her rectum that came on suddenly and went away just as quickly. I asked her to rate her rectal pain on a scale of 1 to 10, with 10 being the worst pain she had ever had, and she said this pain was a "20. Doc, this is worse than anything I have ever had. It's worse than when I slammed my hand in the car door. It's worse than having a baby. It's killing me! I just can't go on like this."

I asked Carrie if she had any fever or chills since her pain began, and she shook her head no. She also denied rectal bleeding, abnormal vaginal bleeding or discharge, or pelvic pain and also denied urinary or fecal incontinance. Her last menstrual period was 1 week ago. She admitted that she quit taking her birth control pills because with this rectal pain, sex was out of the question.

I asked Carrie if she ever had anything like this before, and she shook her head no. I asked what she was doing to manage the pain and she said, "Nothing really works." She had tried Preparation H, thinking she might have a hemorrhoid, a donut pillow her friend gave her, and sitz baths without any significant diminution of symptoms. She went on to say, "Doctor, this may sound nuts, but sometimes when the shooting pain just won't stop, if I insert my finger into my rectum, I can get some relief." I said, "This is useful information and a good clue as to what might be causing your pain."

I asked Carrie to point with one finger to show me where it hurt the most. She pointed to her anus and said, "Doc, you can't see anything. There is nothing there. It's down deep inside. I'm really scared that it's something really bad." I reassured Carrie that we would figure out what was going on and that I would do everything I could to get her better. She gave me a weak smile and said that she hoped so, because she was really worn out getting up 50 times a night to try to go to the bathroom. "Carrie, since this pain has been so hard on you, I have a couple of questions and I want you to really think before answering because they are so important." She said, "Okay, Doc, I will do my best." I said that I knew she would and asked, "Carrie, have you ever felt like life just isn't worth living?" She seemed shocked and then answered, "Doc, if you are asking if this pain makes me want to kill myself, the answer is absolutely not. I have a lot to live for, my boyfriend, my dog Buffy, my job. You don't have to worry about that." "Okay, that's good, Carrie, but I want you to know that you can tell me anything. I make no judgments, no criticism. I'm always here to help." She smiled and said that she really appreciated the concern. "So, next question. Do you feel like you have an excess of worry or stress? You mentioned that there was a lot going on a work." Carrie thought for a moment and admitted that she had been pretty stressed out, but quickly went on to say, "Doctor, the pain is not in my head. It's in my butt." "Okay, that's good to know," I responded. "One last question. Are you being hurt or abused, or have you been hurt and abused in a past relationships or by a stranger or loved one?" Carrie shook her head no, but looked away, making me wonder if something might be going on. "Carrie, this is a place where you can always talk. You can always come for help." She nodded yes and said, "Doctor, just get my tush better and all will be right with the world!"

On physical examination, Carrie was afebrile. Her respirations were 16. Her pulse was 72 and regular. Her blood pressure (BP) was normal at 118/74. Her head, eyes, ears, nose, throat (HEENT) exam was normal, as was her thyroid examination. Her cardiopulmonary examination was negative. Her abdominal examination revealed no abnormal mass or organomegaly. There was no costo-vertebral angle (CVA) tenderness. There was no peripheral edema. Her low back examination was unremarkable. Her lower extremity neurologic examination was completely normal.

I asked Carrie to lie back on the examination table with her knees bent so we could inspect her groin. Inspection of the groin revealed no obvious abnormal mass or inguinal hernia. I again asked Carrie to use one finger to point to the spot that hurt, and she carefully pointed to her anus and again said that the pain was down deep. I asked Carrie if it was okay to do a pelvic and rectal exam and she said that I could do whatever I needed to if it would help get rid of the pain. Visual inspection of the skin and muscosa of the perineum, anus, and external genitalia was normal, with no evidence of trauma or lesions suggestive of herpes or other sexually transmitted diseases. Her rectal and pelvic exam were completely normal, with the stool guaiac negative. Specifically, there were no hemorrhoids, rectal fissures, evidence of trauma, abnormal masses, or rectal pro-lapse on Valsalva. With deep palpation of the levator ani muscles, the paroxysms of pain were triggered, and Carrie asked me to stop. I told Carrie that I had good news. "I didn't find anything bad on the rectal exam." And I had more good news. "I think I know what is wrong and have a pretty good idea of how to fix it." She smiled and said, "Thank God!"

Key Clinical Points—What's Important and What's Not

THE HISTORY

- A history of recent onset of paroxysmal shooting pains deep in the rectum
- No history of gastrointestinal symptoms related to the pain
- No history of gynecologic symptoms related to the pain
- Sleep disturbance
- Admits to increased stress at work
- Pain is localized to the rectum
- No fever or chills
- Denies suicidal ideation
- Denies domestic violence or abuse, but an index of suspicion

THE PHYSICAL EXAMINATION

- The patient is afebrile
- Normal visual inspection of the anus, perineum, external genitalia
- Normal rectal examination
- Stool was guaiac negative
- Normal pelvic examination
- No evidence of rectal prolapse on Valsalva
- Deep palpation of the levator ani muscles triggers the paroxysms of pain
- The neurologic examination is within normal limits

OTHER FINDINGS OF NOTE

- Normal BP
- Normal HEENT examination
- Normal cardiopulmonary examination
- Normal abdominal examination
- No peripheral edema
- No rectal mass or inguinal hernia
- No CVA tenderness

 What Tests Would You Like to Order?

The following tests were ordered:
- Magnetic resonance imaging (MRI) of the pelvis with special attention to the rectal area
- Colonoscopy with special attention to the rectum

TEST RESULTS

MRI of the pelvis is within normal limits. Colonoscopy is completely within normal limits with no evidence of proctitis or other abnormality of the distal colon and rectum.

📋 Clinical Correlation—Putting It All Together

What is the diagnosis?
- Proctalgia fugax

The Science Behind the Diagnosis

ANATOMY OF THE SYMPHYSIS PUBIS

The rectum is the terminal part of the colon, interposed between the sigmoid colon and anus (Figs. 13.1 and 13.2). It connects with the sigmoid colon at the

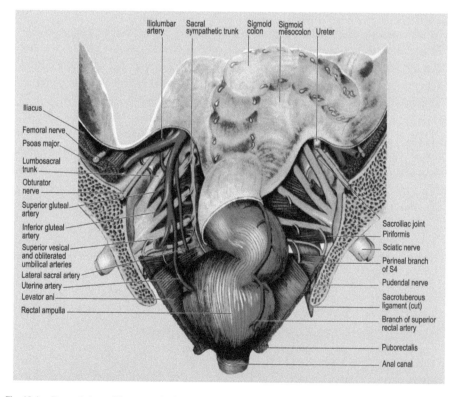

Fig. 13.1 Coronal view of the posterior half of the pelvic cavity, showing the anterior aspect of the rectum. (From Mahadevan V. Anatomy of the rectum and anal canal. *Surgery (Oxford)*. 2020;38[1]:7–11 [Fig. 1].)

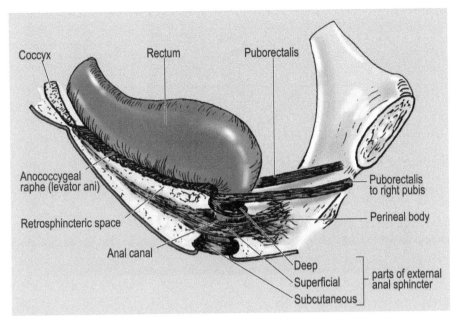

Fig. 13.2 The anorectal junction, puborectalis sling, and external anal sphincter *(right lateral view)*. (From Mahadevan V. Anatomy of the rectum and anal canal. *Surgery (Oxford)*. 2020;38[1]:7–11 [Fig. 2].)

level of S3. The rectum plays an important role in electrolyte and water resorption and as well as a key role in defecation and maintaining fecal continence, as the rectum serves as a terminal reservoir for fecal material. The rectum has a sacral and perineal flexure and has three rectal folds: the superior, middle, and inferior. Blood is supplied to the rectum via the superior, middle, and inferior rectal arteries. Stretch receptors in the rectal walls stimulate the desire to defecate (Fig. 13.3).

CLINICAL SYNDROME

Proctalgia fugax is a disease of unknown cause characterized by paroxysms of rectal pain with pain-free periods between attacks. The pain-free periods between attacks can last seconds to minutes. Similar to cluster headache, spontaneous remissions of the disease occur and may last weeks to years. Proctalgia fugax is more common in women and occurs with greater frequency in patients with irritable bowel syndrome.

The pain of proctalgia fugax is sharp or gripping and severe. Similar to other urogenital focal pain syndromes, such as vulvodynia and prostadynia, the causes remain obscure. Stress and sitting for prolonged periods often increase the frequency and intensity of attacks of proctalgia fugax. Patients often feel an

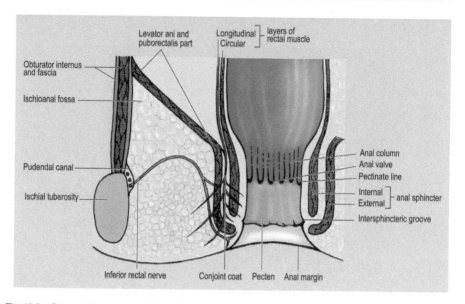

Fig. 13.3 Schematic coronal section of the anal canal and right ischioanal fossa. (From Mahadevan V. Anatomy of the rectum and anal canal. *Surgery (Oxford)*. 2020;38[1]:7–11 [Fig. 3].)

urge to defecate with the onset of the paroxysms of pain (Fig. 13.4). Depression often accompanies the pain of proctalgia fugax but is not thought to be the primary cause. The symptoms of proctalgia fugax can be so severe as to limit the patient's ability to perform activities of daily living.

SIGNS AND SYMPTOMS

The physical examination of a patient with proctalgia fugax is usually normal. The patient may be depressed or appear anxious. Rectal examination is normal, although deep palpation of the surrounding musculature may trigger paroxysms of pain. The patient often reports an ability to abort the attack of pain by placing a finger in the rectum. Bland rectal suppositories also may interrupt the attacks.

TESTING

Similar to the physical examination, testing in patients with proctalgia fugax is usually normal. Because of the risk for overlooking rectal malignancy that may be responsible for pain that may be attributed to a benign cause, by necessity proctalgia fugax is a diagnosis of exclusion. Rectal examination is mandatory in all patients thought to have proctalgia fugax. Sigmoidoscopy or colonoscopy is strongly recommended in such patients with biopsy of suspicious lesions and to

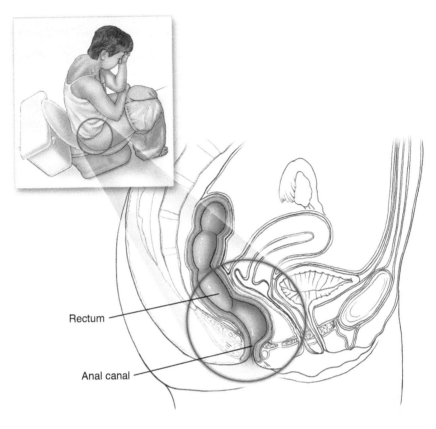

Rectum

Anal canal

Fig. 13.4 Proctalgia fugax is a disease of unknown cause characterized by paroxysms of rectal pain with pain-free periods between attacks. (From Waldman SD. *Atlas of Uncommon Pain Syndromes*. 4th ed. Philadelphia: Saunders; 2020: Fig. 99-1.)

TABLE 13.1 ■ **Signs and Symptoms of Sexually Transmitted Proctitis**

Inflammed muscoa
Bleeding
Purulent exudate
Mucoid exudate
Ulceration
Positive groove sign: enlarged femoral and inguinal lymph nodes separated by inguinal ligament
Strictures
Fistulae
Fissures

aid in the diagnosis of suspected rectal involvement of ulcerative colitis/proctitis. Testing of the stool for occult blood is indicated, as is testing for sexually transmitted proctitis if signs and symptoms are present, with common causative agents including herpes, syphilis, gonorrhea, and chlamydia (Table 13.1). Screening

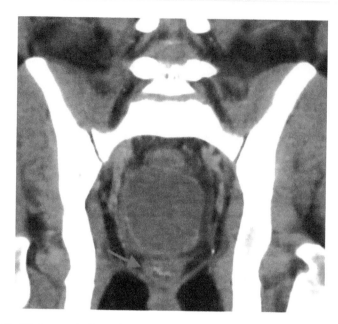

Fig. 13.5 Perirectal abscess *(red arrow)* seen on computed tomography scan. (From Lee M, Izzy M, Ho S. Novel use of fully covered self-expandable metal stent for drainage of perirectal abscess. A case series. *Arab J Gastroenterol.* 2017;18[2]:122–125.)

laboratory studies, consisting of a complete blood cell count, automated chemistries, and erythrocyte sedimentation rate, should be performed. MRI, ultrasound imaging, or computed tomography (CT) of the pelvis should be considered in all patients with proctalgia fugax to rule out occult pathology (Figs. 13.5 and 13.6). If psychological problems are suspected or the patient has a history of sexual abuse, psychiatric evaluation is indicated concurrent with laboratory and radiographic testing.

DIFFERENTIAL DIAGNOSIS

As mentioned previously, because of the risk for overlooking serious pathology of the anus and rectum, proctalgia fugax must be a diagnosis of exclusion. The clinician first must rule out rectal malignancy to avoid disaster. Proctitis and sexually transmitted diseases can mimic the pain of proctalgia fugax and can be diagnosed on sigmoidoscopy or colonoscopy. Hemorrhoids usually manifest with bleeding associated with pain and can be distinguished from proctalgia fugax on physical examination. Prostadynia sometimes may be confused with proctalgia fugax, but the pain is more constant, more dull, and aching.

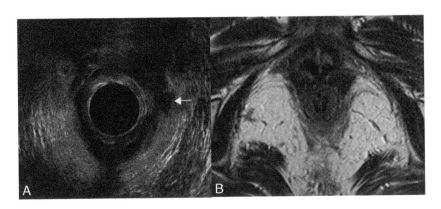

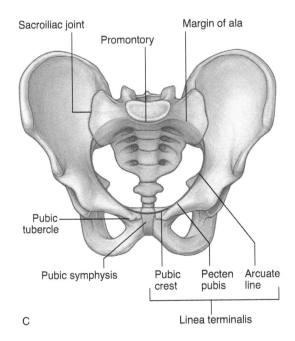

Fig. 13.6 (A) A T3 low rectal tumor, with its radial margin indicated by the arrow in endorectal ultra-sound image. (B) The tumor is poorly visualized by magnetic resonance imaging (MRI) in an axial obli-que T2 high-resolution series. (C) The symphysis pubis. (D) The symphysis pubis. At level 2, the anterior *(arrowheads)* and posterior aponeurosis *(arrow)* are seen. Note pyramidalis muscles in between *(asterisks)*. (E) At level 3, the bulk of the adductor longus tendons is seen *(AL)* inserting on the pubic bone *(Pu)* and cross-connecting via the anterior pubic ligament *(arrow)*. (A–B, From Tsai C, Hague C, Xiong W, et al. Evaluation of endorectal ultrasound (ERUS) and MRI for prediction of circum-ferential resection margin (CRM) for rectal cancer. *Am J Surg.* 2017;213[5]:936–942 [Fig. 5]; C, Vodušek D, Boller F. *Handbook of Clinical Neurology*, vol. 130. Amsterdam: Elsevier; 2015:39–60 [Fig. 2]; D–E, De Maeseneer M, Forsyth R, Provyn S, et al. MR imaging-anatomical-histological evalua-tion of the abdominal muscles, aponeurosis, and adductor tendon insertions on the pubic symphysis: a cadaver study. *Eur J Radiol.* 2019;1113:107–113 [Fig. 3].)

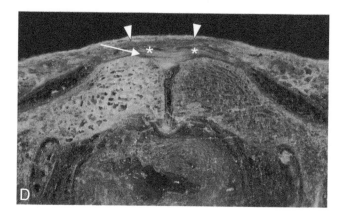

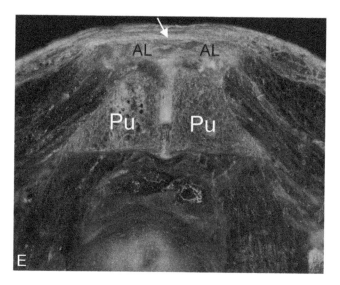

Fig. 13.6 (Continued).

TREATMENT

Initial treatment of proctalgia fugax should include a combination of simple analgesics and nonsteroidal antiinflammatory drugs or cyclooxygenase-2 inhibitors. If these medications do not control the symptoms adequately, a tricyclic antidepressant or gabapentin should be added. Traditionally, tricyclic antidepressants have been a mainstay in the palliation of pain secondary to proctalgia fugax. Controlled studies have shown the efficacy of amitriptyline for this indication. Other tricyclic antidepressants, including nortriptyline and desipramine, also have been shown to be clinically useful. This class of drugs is associated with significant anticholinergic side effects, including dry mouth, constipation, sedation, and urinary retention. These drugs should be used with caution in the elderly and in patients with glaucoma, cardiac arrhythmia, and prostatism.

To minimize side effects and encourage compliance, the primary care physician should start amitriptyline or nortriptyline at a 10-mg dose at bedtime. The dose can be titrated upward to 25 mg at bedtime, as side effects allow. Upward titration of dosage in 25-mg increments can be done each week as side effects allow. Even at lower doses, patients generally report a rapid improvement in sleep disturbance and begin to experience some pain relief in 10 to 14 days. If the patient does not experience any improvement in pain as the dose is being titrated upward, the addition of gabapentin alone or in combination with nerve blocks of the intercostal nerves with local anesthetics, steroid, or both is recommended. Selective serotonin reuptake inhibitors, such as fluoxetine, also have been used to treat the pain of diabetic neuropathy; although better tolerated than the tricyclic antidepressants, they seem to be less efficacious.

If antidepressant compounds are ineffective or contraindicated, gabapentin is a reasonable alternative. Gabapentin should be started with a 300-mg dose at bedtime for 2 nights. The patient should be cautioned about potential side effects, including dizziness, sedation, confusion, and rash. The drug is increased in 300-mg increments, given in equally divided doses over 2 days as side effects allow, until pain relief is obtained or a total dose of 2400 mg daily is reached. At this point, if the patient has experienced partial pain relief, blood values are measured, and the drug is carefully titrated upward using 99-mg tablets. More than 3600 mg daily rarely is required. Clinical reports suggest that the inhalation of salambutol may provide symptomatic relief. Local application of heat and cold also may be beneficial to provide symptomatic relief of the pain of proctalgia fugax. The use of bland rectal suppositories may help provide symptomatic relief. For patients who do not respond to these treatment modalities, injection of the peroneal nerves or caudal epidural nerve block using a local anesthetic and steroid may be a reasonable next step. Ultrasound guidance may improve the accuracy of needle placement and decrease the incidence of needle-related complications. Anecdotal reports indicate that calcium channel blockers, topical nitroglycerin, low dose intravenous lidocaine, and inhalation of albuterol provide symptomatic relief of the pain of proctalgia fugax.

HIGH-YIELD TAKEAWAYS

- The patient's symptomatology was not associated with antecedent trauma or any obvious somatic illness.
- The pain was paroxysmal, with pain-free episodes.

(Continued)

- The pain was located deep in the rectum and sharp in character.
- The patient admitted to increased stress at work.
- The patient's pain was localized to the rectum and does not radiate.
- There were no associated gynecologic, urologic, and gastrointestinal symptoms.
- The patient denied domestic violence or abuse, but index of suspicion must remain high in patients with proctalgia fugax.
- The patient was afebrile, making an acute infectious etiology unlikely.
- All testing was negative.

Suggested Readings

Budak MJ, Oliver TB. There's a hole in my symphysis—a review of disorders causing widening, erosion, and destruction of the symphysis pubis. *Clin Radiol.* 2013;68(2): 173–180.

Glasser JG. Case report: osteitis/osteomyelitis pubis simulating acute appendicitis. *Int J Surg Case Rep.* 2018;53:269–272.

Waldman SD. Injection technique for osteitis pubis. In: *Atlas of Pain Management Injection Techniques.* 4th ed. Philadelphia: Elsevier; 2017:458–461.

Waldman SD. Osteitis pubis. In: *Pain Review.* 2nd ed. Philadelphia: Elsevier; 2017: 296–297.

Waldman SD. Proctalgia fugax. In: *Atlas of Common Pain Syndromes.* 4th ed. Philadelphia: Elsevier; 2017:311–314.

Waldman SD. Proctalgia fugax and other abnormalities of the pubic symphysis. In: *Waldman's Comprehensive Atlas of Diagnostic Ultrasound of Painful Conditions.* Philadelphia: Kluwer Wolters; 2016:640–646.

Waldman SD, Campbell RSD. Anatomy: special imaging considerations of the sacroiliac joint and pelvis. In: *Imaging of Pain.* Philadelphia: Elsevier; 2011:192–196.

Meredith Grace

A 32-Year-Old Female With Right Ill-Defined Low Back and Buttock Pain

- Learn the common causes of sacroiliac pain.
- Develop an understanding of the unique anatomy of the sacroiliac joint.
- Develop an understanding of the causes of sacroiliac joint arthritis.
- Learn the clinical presentation of sacroiliac joint pain.
- Learn how to use physical examination to identify pathology of the sacroiliac joint.
- Develop an understanding of the treatment options for sacroiliac joint pain.
- Learn the appropriate testing options to help diagnose sacroiliac joint pain.
- Learn to identify red flags in patients who present with sacroiliac pain.
- Develop an understanding of the role of interventional pain management in the treatment of sacroiliac pain.

Meredith Grace

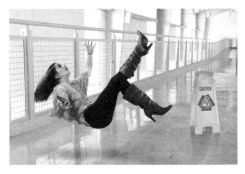

Meredith Grace is a 32-year-old secretary with the chief complaint of, "I've had low back and butt pain since I slipped and fell at the airport." Meredith went on to say that she wouldn't have bothered coming in, but the pain was interfering with her Pilates class. I asked Meredith if anything like this has happened before. She shook her head and said, "Absolutely not. I'm in great shape, but I won't be if you don't get me better. This pain is really wearing me out, and the heating pad and pain pills just aren't doing the job. Doc, I wouldn't complain, but I have to exercise. I usually get up at 5:30 each morning for my Pilates, but I can barely get moving in the morning because my sleep is all jacked up because it hurts every time I roll over on my right side. Can you just give me a quick shot of something to get me back on track? I really need to get back to my routine."

I asked Meredith about any antecedent trauma to the right sacroiliac joint prior to her slip and fall and she said no, that she wouldn't have fallen if she hadn't been in a hurry, and then there were the damn high heel boots and the wet floor. "After all," she said, "my balance is great from all the yoga I do." I asked Meredith to point with one finger to show me where it hurt the most. She pointed to the area of the right sacroiliac joint but noted that it was not well localized. I asked her if the pain radiated anywhere else and she said that sometimes it goes down into the area just below her right buttock, but it didn't go below the knee. Meredith denied any other gynecologic symptoms, blood in her urine, or bowel or bladder symptomatology. Her last menstrual period was about 10 days ago. She was on oral contraceptives.

On physical examination, Meredith was afebrile. Her respirations were 18 and her pulse was 74 and regular. Her blood pressure (BP) was normal at 122/74. Her head, eyes, ears, nose, throat (HEENT) exam was normal, as was her cardiopulmonary examination. Her thyroid was normal. Her abdominal examination revealed no abnormal mass or organomegaly. There was no costovertebral angle (CVA) tenderness. There was no peripheral edema. Her low back examination was unremarkable. I did a rectal exam and pelvic, which were both normal. Visual inspection of the area over the right sacroiliac joint revealed resolving ecchymosis. The area overlying the right sacroiliac joint was cool to touch. Palpation of the right sacroiliac joint revealed moderate diffuse tenderness, with no obvious effusion. I performed a Stork test, which was positive, as were the Yeoman and Van Durson tests (Figs. 14.1 and 14.2). The left sacroiliac

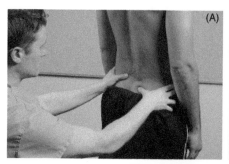
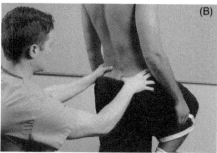
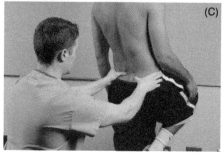

Fig. 14.1 The Stork test for sacroiliac joint pain and dysfunction. (A) The Stork test: The patient is placed in the standing position with the examiner seated behind the patient. The examiner places one thumb on the patient's posterior superior iliac spine and the other thumb on the base of the sacrum. (B) The Stork test: The patient is then asked to flex the hip and knee on the nonpainful side to at least 90 degrees while standing on the contralateral leg. (C) The Stork test: If there is no sacroiliac dysfunction, as the patient flexes the hip and knee, the thumb on the patient's posterior superior iliac spine of the flexed leg will drop as the ilium rotates in a dorsocaudal direction to brace the pelvis to aid the other leg in receiving the full weight of the upper body. (From Waldman SD. *Physical Diagnosis of Pain: An Atlas of Signs and Symptoms*. 3rd ed. St Louis: Elsevier; 2016: Figs. 166-1–166-3.)

joint examination was normal, as was examination of her other major joints. A careful neurologic examination of the upper and lower extremities revealed there was no evidence of peripheral, entrapment neuropathy, or radiculopathy. The deep tendon reflexes were all normal and there were no pathologic reflexes.

Key Clinical Points—What's Important and What's Not

THE HISTORY

- A history of acute trauma to the right sacroiliac joint after a slip and fall
- No history of previous significant sacroiliac pain
- Pain in the area of the right sacroiliac joint radiating into the base of the right buttock
- Pain is not well localized
- Pain does not radiate below the knee
- Increased pain with standing, walking, and taking large steps

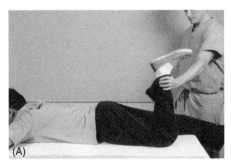
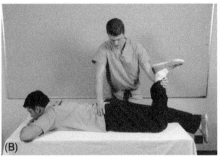
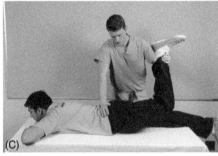

Fig. 14.2 The Yeoman test for sacroiliac joint pain and dysfunction. (A) The Yeoman test: With the patient in prone position, the affected leg is flexed back toward the buttock to 90 degrees. (B) The Yeoman test: The examiner then displaces the ipsilateral ilium with firm downward pressure. (C) The Yeoman test: The examiner then extends the ipsilateral hip. (From Waldman SD. *Physical Diagnosis of Pain: An Atlas of Signs and Symptoms*. 3rd ed. St Louis: Elsevier; 2016: Figs. 166-1–166-3.)

- No fever or chills
- No bowel or bladder symptomatology
- Sleep disturbance

THE PHYSICAL EXAMINATION

- The patient is afebrile
- Resolving ecchymosis over the right sacroiliac joint
- Palpation of right sacroiliac joint reveals moderate diffuse tenderness
- No point tenderness
- No increased temperature of the painful areas
- Positive Yeoman and Van Durson tests (see Figs. 14.1 and 14.2)
- Normal rectal and pelvic examinations

OTHER FINDINGS OF NOTE

- Normal BP
- Normal HEENT examination

- Normal cardiovascular examination
- Normal pulmonary examination
- Normal abdominal examination
- No peripheral edema
- No groin mass or inguinal hernia
- No CVA tenderness
- Normal upper and extremity neurologic examination, motor and sensory examination
- Examination of joints other than the right sacroiliac joint were normal

What Tests Would You Like to Order?

The following tests were ordered:
- Plain radiographs of the right sacroiliac joint

TEST RESULTS

The plain radiographs of the right sacroiliac joint revealed no evidence of arthritis, fracture, or other abnormality (Fig. 14.3).

Clinical Correlation—Putting It All Together

What is the diagnosis?
- Sacroiliac joint pain

The Science Behind the Diagnosis

ANATOMY OF THE HIP JOINTS

The sacroiliac joint is a bicondylar synovial joint that is formed by the articulation between the sacrum and ilium (Fig. 14.4). The articular surface of the sacrum is covered with hyaline cartilage, with the articular surface of the ilium covered with fibrocartilage. These articular surfaces have corresponding elevations and depressions, which give the joints their irregular appearance on radiographs (Fig. 14.5). The strength of the sacroiliac joint comes primarily from the posterior and interosseous ligaments, rather than from the bony articulations (Fig. 14.6). The sacroiliac joints bear the weight of the trunk and are thus subject to the development of strain and arthritis. As the joint ages, the intraarticular space narrows, making intraarticular injection more challenging. The ligaments and the sacroiliac joint itself receive their innervation from L3 to S3 nerve roots, with L4 and L5 providing the greatest

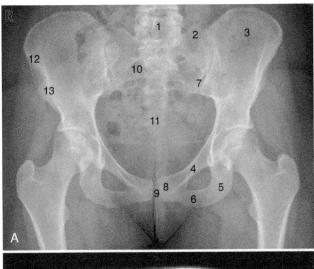

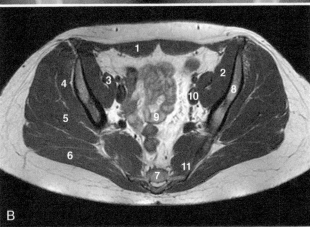

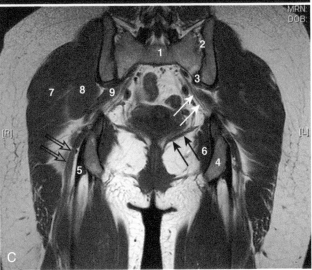

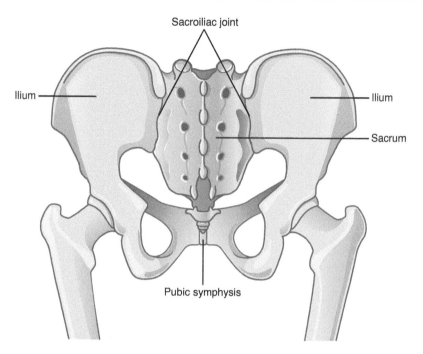

Fig 14.4 The anatomy of the sacroiliac joint. (From Waldman SD. *Atlas of Interventional Pain Management*. 4th ed. Philadelphia: Saunders; 2015: Fig. 119-4.)

contribution to the innervation of the joint. This diverse innervation may explain the ill-defined nature of sacroiliac pain. The sacroiliac joint has a very limited range of motion, and that motion is induced by changes in the forces placed on the joint by shifts in posture and joint loading.

CLINICAL PRESENTATION

Pain from the sacroiliac joint commonly occurs when lifting in an awkward position that puts strain on the joint, its supporting ligaments, and soft

◀ **Fig 14.3** (A) Anteroposterior radiograph of the pelvis: 1, fifth lumbar vertebra; 2, left sacral ala; 3, iliac bone; 4, superior pubic ramus; 5, ischium; 6, inferior pubic ramus; 7, sacroiliac joint (synovial part); 8, body of the pubic bone; 9, pubic symphysis; 10, first sacral foramen; 11, sacrococcygeal junction; 12, anterosuperior iliac spine; 13, anteroinferior iliac spine. (B) Axial T1-weighted magnetic resonance (MR) image of the pelvis: 1, rectus abdominis; 2, iliacus; 3, psoas major; 4, gluteus minimus; 5, gluteus medius; 6, gluteus maximus; 7, sacrum; 8, iliac bone; 9, small bowel; 10, common iliac vein; 11, piriformis (upper border). (C) Coronal T1-weighted MR image of the pelvis: 1, first sacral segment; 2, upper fibrous part of sacroiliac joint; 3, lower synovial part of sacroiliac joint; 4, ischial tuberosity; 5, hamstring tendon origin; 6, obturator internus; 7, gluteus maximus; 8, gluteus medius; 9, piriformis *(white arrows)*, sacral plexus *(black arrows)*, levator ani muscle *(open black arrows)*, sciatic nerve. (From Waldman SD, Campbell RSD. *Imaging of Pain*. Philadelphia: Saunders; 2011: Fig. 77-1.)

POSTERIOR

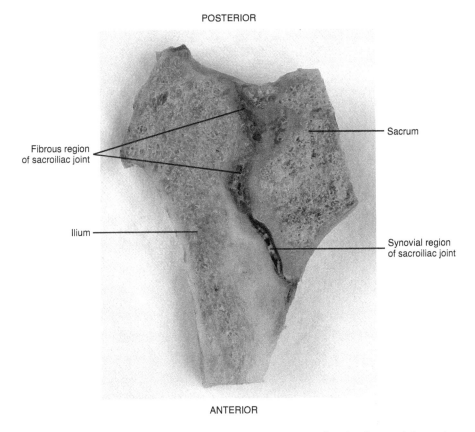

Fig 14.5 The articular surfaces of the sacroiliac joint have corresponding elevations and depressions, which give the joints their irregular appearance on radiographs. (From Waldman SD. *Atlas of Interventional Pain Management*. 4th ed. Philadelphia: Saunders; 2015: Fig. 119-5.)

tissues. The sacroiliac joint is also susceptible to the development of arthritis from various conditions that can damage the joint cartilage. Osteoarthritis is the most common form of arthritis that results in sacroiliac joint pain; rheumatoid arthritis and posttraumatic arthritis are also common causes of sacroiliac joint pain. Less common causes include the collagen vascular diseases such as ankylosing spondylitis, infection, and Lyme disease. Collagen vascular disease generally manifests as polyarthropathy rather than as monoarthropathy limited to the sacroiliac joint, although sacroiliac pain secondary to ankylosing spondylitis responds exceedingly well to the intraarticular injection technique described later. Occasionally, patients present with iatrogenically induced sacroiliac joint dysfunction resulting from overaggressive bone graft harvesting for spinal fusion.

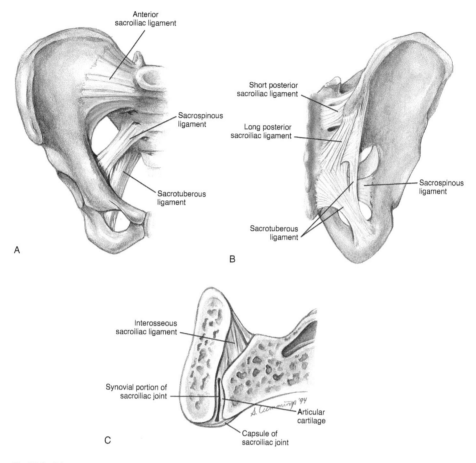

Fig 14.6 Ligaments of the sacroiliac (SI) joint. (A) Anterior view. (B) Posterior view. (C) SI joint in horizontal section. Notice that the capsule of the SI joint is present only anteriorly. (From Cramer GD, Ro CS. The sacrum, sacroiliac joint, and coccyx. In: Cramer GD, Darby SA, eds. *Clinical Anatomy of the Spine, Spinal Cord, and ANS*. 3rd ed. St Louis: Mosby; 2014:312–339.)

SIGNS AND SYMPTOMS

Most patients presenting with sacroiliac joint pain secondary to strain or arthritis complain of pain localized around the sacroiliac joint and upper leg that radiates into the posterior buttock and backs of the legs (Fig. 14.7); the pain does not radiate below the knees. Activity makes the pain worse, whereas rest and heat provide some relief. The pain is constant and is characterized as aching; it may interfere with sleep. On physical examination, the affected sacroiliac joint is tender to palpation. The patient often favors the affected leg and lists toward the unaffected side. Spasm of the lumbar paraspinal musculature is often present, as is limited range

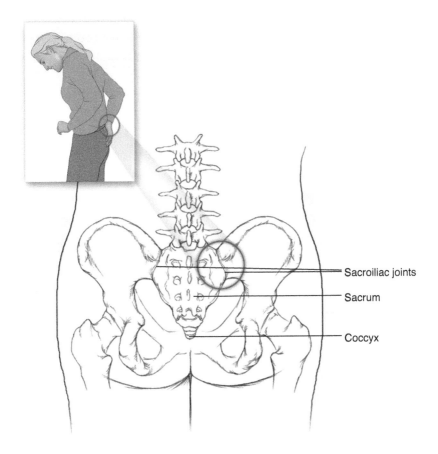

Fig 14.7 Sacroiliac pain is often poorly localized and radiates from the sacroiliac joint into the ipsilateral buttock and upper leg. (From Waldman SD. *Atlas of Common Pain Syndromes*. 4th ed. Philadelphia: Elsevier; 2019: Fig. 87-1.)

of motion of the lumbar spine in the erect position; range of motion improves in the sitting position owing to relaxation of the hamstring muscles.

Patients with pain emanating from the sacroiliac joint exhibit a positive pelvic rock test result. This test is performed by placing the examiner's hands on the iliac crests and the thumbs on the anterior superior iliac spines and then forcibly compressing the patient's pelvis toward the midline. A positive test result is indicated by the production of pain around the sacroiliac joint. Other physical examination tests for sacroiliac joint dysfunction include the Yeoman, Gaenslen, Stork, Piedailu, and Van Durson tests (see Figs. 14.1 and 14.2).

TESTING

Plain radiographs are indicated in all patients who present with sacroiliac pain as other regional pathology may be perceived as sacroiliac pain by the patient (Fig. 14.8). Based on the patient's clinical presentation, additional testing may be indicated, including complete blood cell count, sedimentation rate, and antinuclear antibody testing. Magnetic resonance imaging (MRI) or ultrasound of

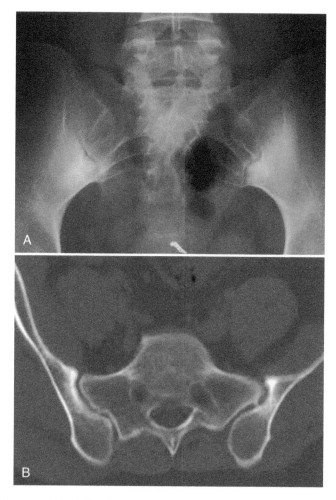

Fig 14.8 (A) Anterioposterior (AP) radiograph of a young postpartum woman with sacroiliac joint (SIJ) pain. Sclerosis confined to the iliac aspect of both SIJs is due to osteitis condensans ilii. (B) An axial computed tomography (CT) scan in a different patient with stress-induced changes due to athletic activity shows the same features of sclerosis of the iliac aspect of the SIJ. Note that in both cases, the joint space is preserved and there is no loss of clarity of the subchondral bone plate and no erosive change. (From Waldman SD, Campbell RSD. *Imaging of Pain*. Philadelphia: Saunders; 2011: Fig. 78-1.)

the sacroiliac is indicated if the diagnosis is in question or infection of the joint is a possibility.

DIFFERENTIAL DIAGNOSIS

Pain emanating from the sacroiliac joint can be confused with low back strain, lumbar bursitis, lumbar fibromyositis, piriformis syndrome, ankylosing spondylitis, inflammatory arthritis, and disorders of the lumbar spinal cord, roots, plexus, and nerves.

TREATMENT

Initial treatment of the pain and functional disability of sacroiliac joint pain includes a combination of nonsteroidal antiinflammatory drugs or cyclooxygenase-2 inhibitors and physical therapy. The local application of heat and cold may also be beneficial. For patients who do not respond to these treatment modalities, injection with local anesthetic and steroid is a reasonable next step.

Injection of the sacroiliac joint is carried out by placing the patient in the supine position and preparing the skin overlying the affected sacroiliac joint space with antiseptic solution. A sterile syringe containing 4 mL of 0.25% preservative-free bupivacaine and 40 mg methylprednisolone is attached to a 25-gauge needle by using strict aseptic technique. The posterior superior spine of the ilium is identified. At this point, the needle is carefully advanced through the skin and subcutaneous tissues at a 45-degree angle toward the affected sacroiliac joint (Fig. 14.9). If bone is encountered, the needle is withdrawn into the subcutaneous tissues and

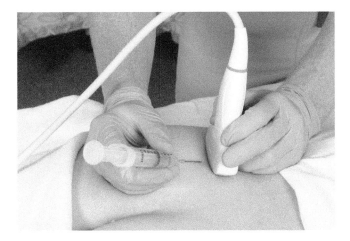

Fig 14.9 Ultrasound-guided sacroiliac joint injection. (From Waldman SD. *Atlas of Interventional Pain Management*. 4th ed. Philadelphia: Saunders; 2015: Fig. 119-22.)

is redirected superiorly and slightly more laterally. After the joint space is entered, the contents of the syringe are gently injected. Little resistance to injection should be felt. If resistance is encountered, the needle is probably in a ligament and should be advanced slightly into the joint space until the injection can proceed without significant resistance. The needle is then removed, and a sterile pressure dressing and ice pack are applied to the injection site. The use of fluoroscopy, computed tomography, and ultrasound guidance may be required in patients in whom the anatomic landmarks are difficult to identify (see Fig. 14.9).

HIGH-YIELD TAKEAWAYS

- The patient is afebrile, making an acute infectious etiology (e.g., septic arthritis) unlikely.
- The patient's symptomatology is the result of acute trauma from a slip and fall.
- The patient's pain is diffuse rather than highly localized, as would be the case with a pathologic process such as ischiogluteal bursitis.
- The pain of sacroiliac joint does not radiate below the knee.
- Physical diagnosis is useful in the diagnosis of sacroiliac joint pain.
- The patient's symptoms are unilateral and involve only one joint, which is more suggestive of a local process than a systemic polyarthropathy.
- Sleep disturbance is common and must be addressed concurrently with the patient's pain symptomatology.
- Plain radiographs will provide high-yield information regarding the joint, but ultrasound imaging and MRI will be more useful in identifying soft tissue pathology.

Suggested Readings

Carvajal-Flechas F, Sarmiento-Monroy JC, Rojas-Villarraga A, et al. Septic sacroiliitis in the late postpartum due to Escherichia coli. *Rev Colombiana Reumatol (English Edition)*. 2016;23(2):131−136.

Petrides S. Non-inflammatory sacroiliac joint disorders. *Indian J Rheumatol*. 2014;9(2): S54−S63.

Prakash J. Sacroiliac tuberculosis—a neglected differential in refractory low back pain—our series of 35 patients. *J Clin Orthop Trauma*. 2014;5(3):146−153.

Waldman SD. Arthritis pain of the hip. In: *Atlas of Common Pain Syndromes*. 4th ed. Philadelphia: Elsevier; 2019:383−386.

Waldman SD. Intra-articular injection of the sacroiliac joint. In: *Atlas of Pain Management Injection Techniques*. 4th ed. Philadelphia: Elsevier; 2017:429−434.

Waldman SD. Lumbar radiculopathy. In: *Pain Review*. 2nd ed. Philadelphia: Elsevier; 2017:223−224.

Waldman SD. Sacroiliitis and other abnormalities of the sacrococcygeal joint. In: *Waldman's Comprehensive Atlas of Diagnostic Ultrasound of Painful Conditions*. Philadelphia: Kluwer Wolters; 2016:710−716.

Waldman SD. The Yeoman test for sacroiliac pain. In: *Physical Diagnosis of Pain: An Atlas of Signs and Symptoms*. 3rd ed. Philadelphia: Elsevier; 2016:254–255.

Waldman SD, Campbell RSD. Anatomy: special imaging considerations of the sacroiliac joint and pelvis. In: *Imaging of Pain*. Philadelphia: Elsevier; 2011:192–196.

Waldman SD, Campbell RSD. Sacroiliac joint pain. In: *Imaging of Pain*. Philadelphia: Elsevier; 2011:197–200.

Buddy Johnson

A 32-Year-Old Male With Tailbone Pain Following a Fall off a Ladder

- Learn the common causes of coccygeal pain.
- Develop an understanding of the anatomy of the coccyx.
- Develop an understanding of the causes of coccydynia.
- Develop an understanding of the differential diagnosis of coccygeal pain.
- Learn the clinical presentation of coccydynia.
- Learn how to use physical examination to identify coccydynia.
- Develop an understanding of the treatment options for coccydynia.

Buddy Johnson

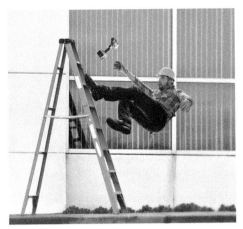

Buddy Johnson is a 32-year-old electrician with the chief complaint of, "Ever since I fell off my ladder, I've had a horrible pain in my tailbone." Buddy stated that a couple of months ago, he was installing a security camera on the outside of a building when he missed a step on his ladder and fell backward and landed right on his tailbone. He said that he's lucky he didn't break his neck, but as he got up he noticed a sharp pain in his tailbone. The pain was so severe that he had a hard time walking back to his truck. Buddy noted that sitting down on his truck seat made the pain much worse. He figured he would get better over the next few days, but it just didn't happen. Sitting became a real problem, as did squatting and climbing a ladder. He tried both ice packs and a heating pad, which provided only minimal relief. He used Extra-strength Tylenol, which he felt took the edge off. "Doctor, this is real pain in the ass. Being an electrician is not a spectator sport. I am up and down my ladder 50 to 60 times a day, and I need to be 100% because I am working with 220 and 440 every day. I can't believe I fell off my ladder. I should know better."

I asked Buddy if he had experienced any pain, numbness, or weakness in his legs since the fall and he just shook his head and replied, "Never. Doc, the pain is all right in my tailbone, and if I push on it—oh boy, the pain goes through the roof!" I asked Buddy how he was sleeping and he said, "Not worth a crap. Every time I roll over, the pain in my tailbone wakes me up. My wife is sleeping in our kid's room because I keep waking her up. The biggest problem is that I can't sit for more than a few minutes without the pain getting so bad that I have to get up. Driving has become a real problem, too. I'm afraid I'm going to lose my job."

I asked Buddy to show me where the pain was and he pointed to his tailbone. "Doc, this is right where the pain is." I asked, "Does the pain radiate anywhere?" Buddy shook his head and said, "It's just the tailbone. I must have broke it or something." I asked Buddy about any fever, chills, or other constitutional symptoms such as weight loss, night sweats, etc., and he shook his head no. He denied any musculoskeletal, systemic symptoms, or bowel or bladder symptoms.

On physical examination, Buddy was afebrile. His respirations were 18, his pulse was 72 and regular, and his blood pressure was 124/76. Buddy's head, eyes, ears, nose, throat (HEENT) exam was normal, as was his thyroid exam. Auscultation of his carotids revealed no bruits, and the pulses in all four extremities were normal. He had a regular rhythm without ectopy. His cardiac exam was otherwise unremarkable. His abdominal examination revealed no abnormal mass or organomegaly. There was no peripheral edema. His low back examination was unremarkable. There was no costovertebral angle (CVA) tenderness. Visual inspection of the right buttock and the skin over his coccyx was unremarkable; specifically, there was no rubor or color and no evidence of ecchymosis. Palpation of the coccyx did not reveal any obvious deformity or abnormal mass, but it caused Buddy to cry out in pain. "Doc, you're right on it. Please don't push that hard." I did a rectal exam, and when I palpated Buddy's coccyx, he came off the table. "Doc, I have had about all the fun I want to with that— enough already!" A careful neurologic examination of both lower extremities was within normal limits. Deep tendon reflexes were physiologic throughout.

Key Clinical Points—What's Important and What's Not

THE HISTORY

- A history of onset of severe coccygeal pain immediately following a fall from a ladder
- The pain is localized to the coccyx
- Sitting or any activities that cause pressure or movement of the coccyx cause pain
- There are no bowel or bladder symptoms
- There is significant sleep disturbance
- No fever or chills

THE PHYSICAL EXAMINATION

- The patient is afebrile
- Marked tenderness to palpation of the coccyx
- Marked pain with movement of the coccyx on rectal examination
- Palpation of the coccyx on rectal examination did not reveal any obvious deformity or abnormal mass
- Normal neurologic examination

OTHER FINDINGS OF NOTE

- Normal HEENT examination
- Normal cardiovascular examination
- Normal pulmonary examination
- Normal abdominal examination
- No peripheral edema

What Tests Would You Like to Order?

The following test was ordered:
- X-ray of the coccyx

TEST RESULTS

X-ray of the coccyx reveals an inline fracture with no obvious displacement (Fig. 15.1).

(a)

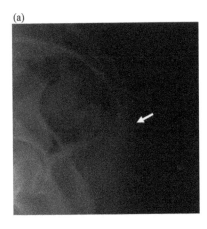

(b)

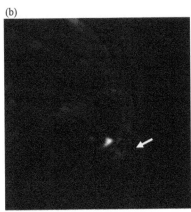

Fig. 15.1 (a) Initial lateral standing coccyx X-ray demonstrating no displacement. *(White arrow)* Disruption of coccyx with inline fracture appearing as normal anatomy. (b) Magnetic resonance imaging of coccyx showing marrow edema *(white arrow)*. (From Dayawansa S, Garrett D, Wong M, et al. Management of coccydynia in the absence of X-ray evidence: case report. *Int J Surg Case Rep.* 2019;54:63–65 [fig. 1].)

Clinical Correlation—Putting It All Together

What is the diagnosis?

- Coccydynia secondary to acute trauma that resulted in a nondisplaced fracture

The Science Behind the Diagnosis

ANATOMY

The five sacral vertebrae are fused together to form the triangular-shaped sacrum (Fig. 15.2). The dorsally convex sacrum inserts in a wedgelike manner between the two iliac bones with superior articulations with the fifth lumbar vertebra and caudad articulations with the coccyx. On the anterior concave surface, there are four pairs of unsealed anterior sacral foramina that allow passage of the

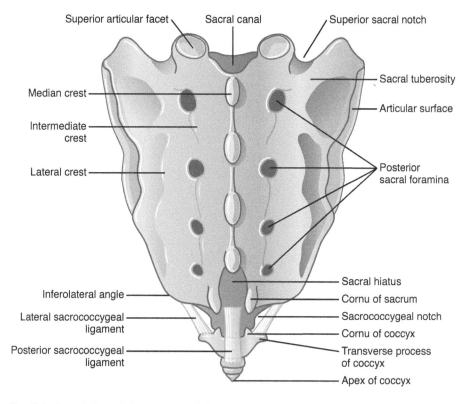

Fig. 15.2 Dorsal view of the anatomy of the sacrum and coccyx. (From Waldman SD. *Atlas of Interventional Pain Management.* 4th ed. Philadelphia: Saunders; 2015: Fig. 105-3.)

anterior rami of the upper four sacral nerves. The posterior sacral foramina are smaller than their anterior counterparts. Leakage of drugs injected into the sacral canal is effectively prevented by the sacrospinal and multifidus muscles. The vestigial bony remnants that are the result of the incomplete fusion of the inferior articular processes of the lower half of the S4, and all of the S5 vertebrae project downward on each side of the sacral hiatus (see Fig. 15.2). These bony projections are called the sacral cornua and represent important clinical landmarks when performing ultrasound-guided caudal epidural nerve block. The U-shaped sacral hiatus is covered posteriorly by the sacrococcygeal ligament, which is also an important clinical landmark when performing ultrasound-guided caudal epidural nerve block. Penetration of the sacrococcygeal ligament provides direct access to the epidural space of the sacral canal. The triangular coccyx is made up of three to five rudimental vertebrae. Its superior surface articulates with the inferior articular surface of the sacrum (Fig. 15.3).

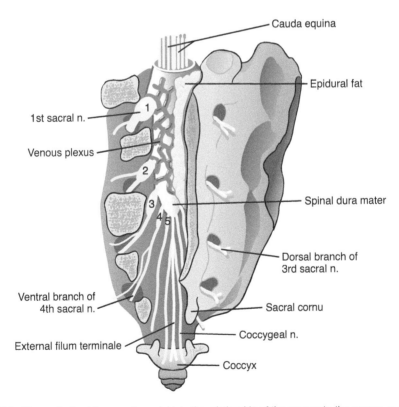

Fig. 15.3 The contents of the sacral canal. Note the relationship of the sacrum to the coccyx. *n*, nerve. (From Waldman SD. *Atlas of Interventional Pain Management.* 4th ed. Philadelphia: Saunders; 2015: Fig. 105-4.)

CLINICAL SYNDROME

Coccydynia is a common syndrome characterized by pain localized to the tailbone that radiates into the lower sacrum and perineum (Fig. 15.4). Coccydynia affects females more frequently than males. It occurs most commonly after direct trauma from a kick or a fall directly onto the coccyx. Coccydynia can also occur after a difficult vaginal delivery (Table 15.1). The pain of coccydynia is thought to be the result of strain of the sacrococcygeal ligament or occasionally, fracture of the coccyx. Less commonly, arthritis of the sacrococcygeal joint can result in coccydynia (Fig. 15.5).

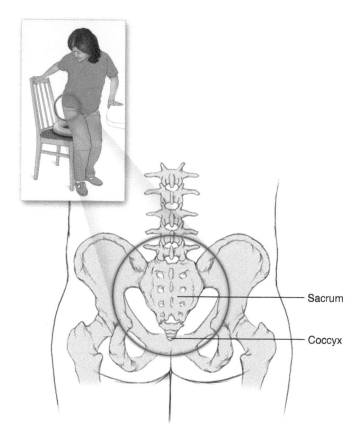

Sacrum

Coccyx

Fig. 15.4 Coccydynia is a common syndrome characterized by pain localized to the tailbone that radiates into the lower sacrum and perineum. (From Waldman SD. *Atlas of Common Pain Syndromes*. 4th ed. Philadelphia: Elsevier; 2019: Fig. 97-1.)

TABLE 15.1 ▪ Etiology of Coccydynia

Postpartum
Traumatic
Degenerative
Idiopathic
Psychosomatic

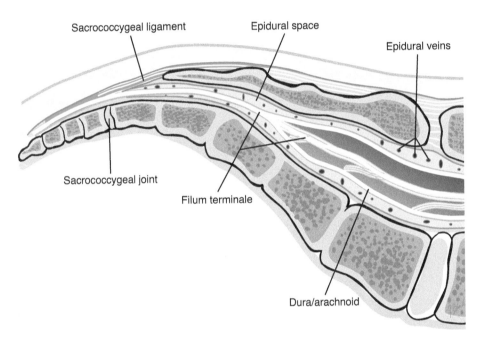

Fig. 15.5 Cross-section of the sacrum and coccyx and the contents. Note the relationship of sacrococcygeal ligament to the coccyx. (From Waldman SD. *Atlas of Interventional Pain Management.* 4th ed. Philadelphia: Saunders 2015: Fig. 105-2.)

SIGNS AND SYMPTOMS

On physical examination, patients exhibit point tenderness over the coccyx; the pain increases with movement of the coccyx. Movement of the coccyx may also cause sharp paresthesias into the rectum, which patients find quite distressing. On rectal examination, the levator ani, piriformis, and coccygeus muscles may feel indurated, and palpation of these muscles may induce severe spasm. Sitting exacerbates the pain of coccydynia, and patients often attempt to sit on one buttock to avoid pressure on the coccyx.

15—TAILBONE PAIN FOLLOWING A FALL OFF A LADDER

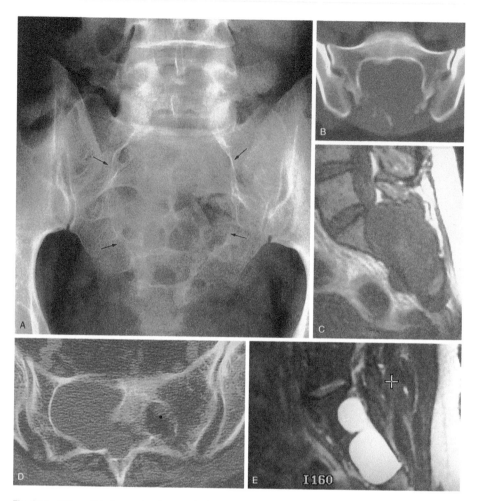

Fig. 15.6 Differential diagnosis of coccydynia. (A–C) Ependymoma. In this 28-year-old woman with low back pain of several years' duration and a normal neurologic examination, routine radiography (A) reveals an osteolytic lesion *(arrows)* in the sacrum. Transaxial computed tomography (CT) scan (B) confirms its central location and posterior extension. Sagittal T1-weighted spin-echo magnetic resonance imaging (C) shows its large size, posterior extension, and low signal intensity. The tumor was of high signal intensity on T2-weighted spin-echo MRI *(not shown)*. Histologic analysis confirmed a myxopapillary ependymoma that did not communicate with the dural sac. (D, E) Meningocele. Transaxial CT scan (D) shows a right-sided sacral lesion distorting the neural foramen. It is sharply delineated, with a sclerotic margin. Sagittal fast spin-echo MRI (E) reveals a lesion of high signal intensity with bone erosion. (From Resnick D. *Diagnosis of Bone and Joint Disorders.* 4th ed. Philadelphia: Saunders; 2002:4018.)

TESTING

Plain radiography is indicated in all patients who present with pain thought to be emanating from the coccyx to rule out occult bony pathology and tumor (Fig. 15.6). Based on the patient's clinical presentation, additional testing may be

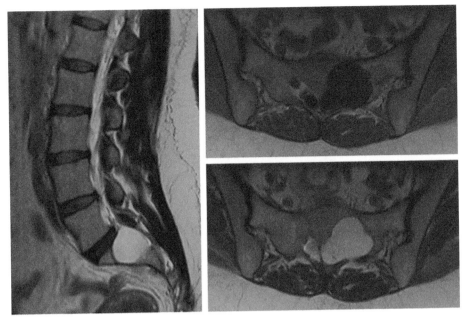

Fig. 15.7 Axial and sagittal T1- and T2-weighted lumbar magnetic resonance images showing a sacral Tarlov cyst. The cyst caused vertebral body remodeling and abnormal dilatation of the S1 left intervertebral foramina. (From Peña E, Llanero M. Painful legs and moving toes syndrome associated with a sacral Tarlov cyst. *Parkinsonism Relat Disord*. 2011;17[8]:645–646.)

TABLE 15.2 ■ **Pathologic Processes That May Cause Coccydynia**

Arthritis
Crystal deposition disease
Ligamentous abnormality
Abnormal coccygeal morphology
Infection
Discogenic disease
Tumor
Pelvic muscle dysfunction
Referred pain

warranted, including a complete blood count, prostate-specific antigen level, erythrocyte sedimentation rate, and antinuclear antibody testing. Magnetic resonance imaging (MRI), computed tomography (CT) scanning, and ultrasound imaging of the pelvis are indicated if occult mass or tumor is suspected (Fig. 15.7). Radionuclide bone scanning may be useful to rule out stress fractures not visible on plain radiographs. Injection of the sacrococcygeal ligament and joint may serve as both a diagnostic and a therapeutic maneuver.

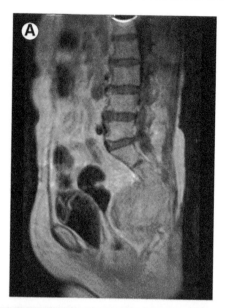

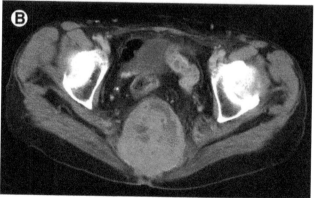

Fig. 15.8 Magnetic resonance imaging (A) and computed tomography findings (B) of a typical sacro-coccygeal chordoma. (From Gronchi A, Casali PG, Olmi P. Sacro-coccygeal chordoma: diagnosis and treatment review. *Sem Colon Rectal Surg.* 2004;15[1]:26–32 [Fig. 1].)

DIFFERENTIAL DIAGNOSIS

Primary pathology of the rectum and anus is occasionally confused with the pain of coccydynia (Table 15.2). Primary tumors or metastatic lesions of the sacrum or coccyx may also present as coccydynia (Fig. 15.8). Proctalgia fugax can be distinguished from coccydynia because movement of the coccyx does not reproduce the pain. Insufficiency fractures of the pelvis or sacrum and pathology of the sacroiliac joints may on occasion mimic coccydynia.

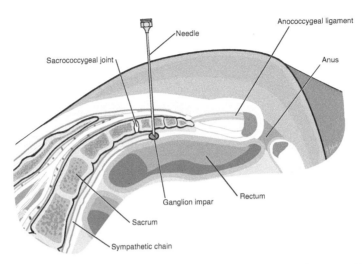

Fig. 15.9 A 3.5-inch spinal needle is inserted between the first and second coccygeal bones and slowly advanced until the needle tip rests just beyond the anterior wall of the coccyx in the precoccygeal space. (From Waldman SD. *Atlas of Interventional Pain Management*. 4th ed. Philadelphia: Saunders; 2015: Fig. 116-4.)

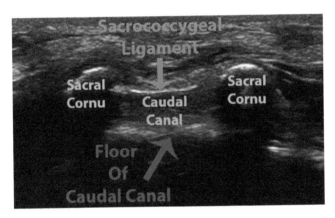

Fig. 15.10 Injection of the sacrococcygeal joint and ligament may serve as a diagnostic and therapeutic maneuver in patients suffering from coccydynia. Ultrasound guidance may improve the accuracy of needle placement. (Courtesy Steven Waldman, MD.)

TREATMENT

Initial treatment of the pain and functional disability associated with coccydynia includes a combination of nonsteroidal antiinflammatory drugs or cyclooxygenase-2 inhibitors and physical therapy. The local application of heat and cold may also be beneficial. Any repetitive activity that may exacerbate the patient's symptoms should be avoided. If the patient is a back sleeper, then sleeping on the side while placing a pillow between the legs may be helpful. For patients who do not respond to these treatment modalities, injection of local anesthetic and methyl-prednisolone in the region of the sacrococcygeal joint and ligament is a reasonable next step. Ganglion impar block with local anesthetic and steroid may also be considered if the pain is thought to be sympathetically mediated (Fig. 15.9). Ultrasound needle guidance will improve the accuracy of needle placement and decrease the incidence of needle-induced complications (Fig. 15.10). Rarely, surgical release of the entrapment is required to obtain relief.

HIGH-YIELD TAKEAWAYS

- The patient is afebrile, making an acute infectious etiology unlikely.
- The patient's symptomatology is most likely due to trauma to the coccyx from a fall from a ladder.
- Physical examination and testing should be focused on identification of other pathologic processes that may mimic the clinical diagnosis of coccydynia.
- The patient exhibits the physical examination findings that are highly suggestive of coccydynia.
- The patient's symptoms are localized.
- Plain radiographs of the coccyx will help identify bony abnormalities of the coccyx, including fractures, dislocations, and osseous tumors.
- Ultrasound imaging, CT scanning, and MRI of the coccyx and pelvis may help identify less common causes of pain in the area of the sacrum and coccyx (e.g., tumor, lipoma, or neural tumors).

Suggested Readings

Fritz J, Chhabra A, Wang KC, et al. Magnetic resonance neurography–guided nerve blocks for the diagnosis and treatment of chronic pelvic pain syndrome. *Neuroimag Clin N Am.* 2014;24(1):211–234.

Waldman SD. Coccydynia. In: *Atlas of Common Pain Syndromes.* 4th ed. Philadelphia, PA: Elsevier; 2017:378–382.

Waldman SD. Coccydynia. In: *Pain Review.* 2nd ed. Philadelphia, PA: Elsevier; 2017:302–303.

Waldman SD. Coccydynia and other abnormalities of the sacrococcygeal joint. In: *Diagnostic Ultrasound of Painful Conditions.* Philadelphia, PA: Lippincott; 2016:703–708.

Waldman SD. Injection technique for coccydynia. In: *Pain Review.* 2nd ed. Philadelphia, PA: Elsevier; 2017:553.

Page numbers followed by 'f' indicate figures, 't' indicate tables, 'b' indicate boxes.

A

B

Groin pain (*Continued*)
    differential diagnosis, 39, 40*f*
    distribution, 36*t*
    testing, 38–39
    treatment, 40–42, 41*f*
  incidence, 144
  injection of, 149*f*
  proximal, 143*f*
  right, 31
  suprapubic pain, 103*f*
  testing, 148
  treatment, 150

H

Hip
  acetabulum, 7
  anatomy, joints, 7, 8*f*
  avascular necrosis, 11*f*
Hip joint
  anatomy, 7, 8*f*, 20–21, 188–190, 190*f*
  arthritis of, 7, 9*f*
  blood supply, 20–21, 22*f*
  magnetic resonance imaging, 21*f*, 25*f*
  osteonecrosis, 20*f*
Hip pain
  avascular necrosis, 17, 20
    and alcohol abuse, 22
    clinical presentation, 21–22
    differential diagnosis, 25–26
    predisposing factors, 23*t*
    and steroids, 22
    treatment, 27
    ultrasound image, 26*f*
  causes, 12*t*
  diagnosis, 20
  differential diagnosis, 9, 12*t*
  left, 17
    magnetic resonance imaging, 21*f*
  posterior, 69. *See also* Ischial bursitis

N
Numbness, lateral thigh, 45–46

O
Obturator nerve
  anatomy, 127–130, 128*f*, 129*f*
  clinical syndrome, 130–131
  entrapment of, 132*f*
  neuralgia
    differential diagnosis, 134
    testing of, 132–133, 133*f*
    treatment, 134–135
  neuropathy, 131
  sensory distribution, 127–130, 131*f*
Osteitis pubis pain, suprapubic pain, 97*f*, 101, 103*b*
  isotope bone scan, 105*f*
  needle placement for injection, 105*f*, 106*f*
Osteoarthritis
  right hip pain, 5, 6*f*, 10*f*
  sacroiliac joint pain, 190–191
Osteonecrosis, femoral head, 24*f*
Osteophyte formation, right hip pain, 6*f*

P
Parethesias, 118–120
Patrick (FABER) test, 4–5, 4*f*
Pelvic pain, 95, 171
Perirectal abscess, 178*f*
Piedailu tests, sacroiliac joint
        pain, 193
Pins-and-needles sensation, lateral thigh, 45–46
Piriformis muscle, 159
Piriformis syndrome, 159–162
  differential diagnosis, 167
  injection technique for, 166*f*
  sciatic nerve in, 164*f*
  signs and symptoms, 162, 163*f*, 164*f*
  testing, 154*f*, 155, 163–166
  treatment, 167